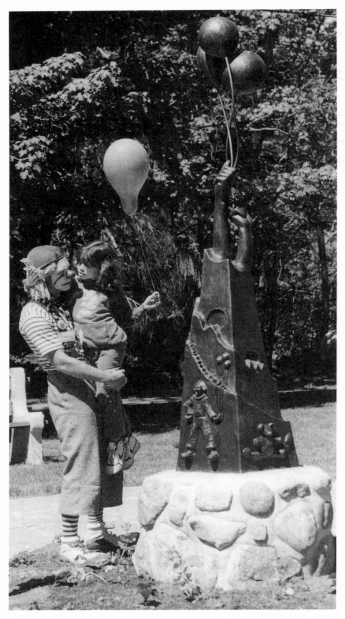

"Crossroads the Clown" and a camper visit the Statue Garden. Photo by Stephen D. Cannerelli.

FOR THE LOVE OF TEDDI

The Story Behind Camp Good Days and Special Times

The 2001 Edition

Lou Buttino

PRAEGER

Westport, Connecticut
London

Library of Congress Cataloging-in-Publication Data

Buttino, Lou.
    For the love of Teddi : the story behind Camp Good Days and Special Times / Lou
Buttino—2001 ed. [rev.].
        p.   cm.
    Includes bibliographical references and index.
    ISBN 0–275–97341–7 (alk. paper)
        1. Mervis, Teddi—Health.   2. Brain—Cancer—Patients—Biography.   3. Tumors in
children—Patients—Biography.   4. Camp Good Days and Special Times (N.Y.).   5.
Recreational therapy for children.   I. Title.
    RC280.B7 M463 2001
    362.1′9892994—dc21
    [B]   00–065570

British Library Cataloguing in Publication Data is available.

Library of Congress Catalog Card Number: 00–065570
ISBN: 0–275–97341–7

First published in 2001

Praeger Publishers, 88 Post Road West, Westport, CT 06881
An imprint of Greenwood Publishing Group, Inc.
www.praeger.com

Printed in the United States of America

The paper used in this book complies with the
Permanent Paper Standard issued by the National
Information Standards Organization (Z39.48–1984).

10 9 8 7 6 5 4 3 2 1

Contents

Preface

The idea for this book came on a cold February day in 1982 as I sat alone with Teddi in her room on the fourth floor of Strong Memorial Hospital in Rochester, New York. As I looked at Teddi, lying there in a deep coma, I couldn't help but think back on all that happened during the almost three years since she had first been diagnosed as having a malignant brain tumor. Now, more than a decade later, the reach of Teddi's life has extended nationally and even internationally.

For the Love of Teddi shows how our family tried to make something positive out of the devastation of childhood cancer. It started as an attempt to bring childhood cancer out of the dark ages. Now we have built the largest, and one of the most unique organizations in the world which deals specifically with childhood cancer. Camp Good Days and Special Times is an obligation fulfilled—an obligation adults and the healthy have to afflicted children.

In 1982, when Teddi died, childhood cancer was the second leading cause of death in children—followed only by accidents. The statistics have not changed much. What has changed, however, is the hearts and minds of literally thousands of others—children, brothers and sisters, parents, grandparents, sports and entertainment celebrities, politicians and so many more, here and around the globe—who have become part of Teddi's story.

In preparing this book, Lou Buttino conducted more than fifty interviews to ensure that Teddi's story would be told honestly and from many points of view—that of family, doctors, nurses, classmates, friends, other children with cancer, clergy and neighbors. *For the Love of Teddi* is a real life drama—an American love story. But most of all it is an inspiration of how something good and enduring can come from an experience as uniquely tragic as the death of a child.

I hope as you read this book it will be as inspiring to you as Teddi's short life was to all of us who knew and loved her. Though she is missed deeply, her presence is felt in the faces and words of so many I have met and heard from over the years. And now you join her circle of friends.

—Gary H. Mervis

PART I

A World Comes Apart

1

That First Night

April 18, 1979, started off as a beautiful spring day. Winter had suddenly shrugged off its long stay, like an overcoat, and flowers, shrubs, and trees burst forth with new life.

Sheri Mervis, in her early thirties, was at work that day. Employed by the Monroe County Sheriff's Department, she was part of a security team responsible for safety in the courtroom and the transfer of prisoners. Gary, her husband, also in his early thirties, spent part of the day at the Mohawk Printing Company where he worked as director of marketing and public relations. He was a part-time employee of the New York State Legislature as well. Smart, a good strategist, Gary was making a name for himself in local and state Republican politics.

The couple married young and now had three children: Tod, 13; Kim, 11; and Teddi, 9. Sheri, with blonde hair and blue eyes, was more reserved than her dark-haired, outgoing husband, whom all the children resembled.

It was the start of Easter vacation and Tod had gone off with some friends for the day. Kim and Teddi, along with their friend Chrissy, had stayed home and played at dressing up in Sheri's clothes. The three caked themselves with make-up and looked more like clowns than beauty queens with the generous coating of lipstick they painted on each other. After spraying themselves with perfume, they headed for the driveway where they pranced, danced, and sang to the music of a radio blaring from the garage.

It was going to be a hard day for Teddi because her mother decided it was time for Kim to develop friendships of her own and have experiences independent of Teddi. Teddi and Kim had done practically everything together to that point but their mother, having grown up with a younger sister, thought it best to begin separating the two. And so Kim was going to spend that night with her friend Chrissy. Teddi was not invited to come along.

Late in the afternoon, the three girls went inside to wash up and change. Chrissy's mother, Irene, was to arrive shortly.

Irene Matichyn, in her thirties like most of the Mervis friends, had come to know the family through her political work with Gary. Blunt and often irreverent, she had been Gary's assistant at the Republican State Assembly Office and then took over his job when he went on to become an assistant to Assemblyman Jim Nagle of East Rochester. Over the past few years Irene and Sheri, like their daughters, had developed a strong friendship.

Kim and Chrissy climbed into the car in silence. Irene waved and called out to Teddi. "She was crying her heart out," Irene recalled. "I was taking her sister and we didn't want her. Nobody cared about her."

Teddi and her mother ate supper together that night. Teddi wasn't talkative, nor did she show much enthusiasm for doing anything in particular. She did complain about her eye twitching and her mother rubbed it for awhile. Being active herself, Sheri knew about muscle spasms. Though Teddi liked to read, this night her mother read to her.

Gary had tickets to the Red Wing opener, Rochester's minor league team, and had gone to the ball game with a friend. He stopped home briefly after the game, on his way to the State Assembly Office. It was about 6:30.

Though home briefly, Gary remarked about Teddi's unusually subdued mood. His wife reminded him about this being the first time Teddi was left behind. Gary shook his head, and then left.

Later in the evening, as Sheri and her daughter sat on the couch, Teddi said: "Mommy, my teddy bear doesn't have a name."

Teddi's bear was brown, with shiny black eyes. Its red felt mouth was partially gone, and the area around its nose and mouth was threadbare from wear. It had been Teddi's first bear.

Sheri, a matter-of-fact kind of person, didn't skip a beat in answering. "Of course it has a name," she said. "It's 'Teddy Bear.' "

"Oh, Mommy," said the girl, "that's a boy's name. My bear's a girl."

Her mother thought it over for a minute and then suggested they call the bear "Teddietta."

Teddi smiled and seemed satisfied, and her mother returned to reading out loud to her. Sheri glanced up now and then and saw in the reflective stare of her daughter that the one thing in the world she needed most now was a friend of her own. 'Teddietta will have to do for now,' Sheri thought to herself.

"My eye's still twitching," Teddi interrupted.

Her mother rubbed it again, questioning: "It stopped for a while, though, didn't it, Teddi?"

Teddi didn't think it had. Her mother thought perhaps the child had not noticed.

The Mervis children were allowed to go to bed at whatever time they chose—there were no curfews unless a child had been unusually bad. Teddi was seldom a bad child, though. She was the helper around the house, a giver, somebody who smiled a lot and seemed to enjoy life immensely.

Teddi decided it was bedtime and went to her room to get changed. Sheri put the book away, and Tod arrived home. Shortly afterward, Gary arrived home, too.

The couple talked about the day's events and then the focus became Teddi, how quiet she had been, how hard it must have been for her to see Kim leave without her.

Sheri left to see how Teddi was doing and was shocked to find Teddi with all her clothes on, standing up, her left eye and left arm twitching erratically.

"What are you doing, honey?" Sheri asked, alarmed but trying to keep control.

"Nothing, Mommy," Teddi answered.

"What do you mean you're doing nothing. You're twitching."

"But I can't help it," Teddi answered.

Sheri again asked Teddi what was wrong, but Teddi shrugged.

"Stop it, Teddi!" Sheri blurted. "You're scaring me!"

Teddi said she couldn't stop.

"I'm going to call an ambulance to take you to the hospital if you don't stop," her mother then said, thinking that if Teddi was faking, a threat like that would put an end to it.

The child nodded assent. "Okay, Mommy," she said. "Please do that."

Her own heart pounding now, Sheri went to her daughter, kneeling down beside her. She held her for a moment. "Come into the living room, Teddi," she whispered. "We'll sit you down."

Both started walking toward the living room but Teddi was too wobbly. Her face also began to twitch. Her eye and arm were still twitching. Sheri picked up her daughter and carried her to the couch in the living room. Hearing troubled voices, Tod came from his room. Gary came quickly as well.

All three took turns trying to get the twitching to stop. Gary thought that maybe she was having a small epileptic seizure. He had worked with children as a recreation supervisor and had seen symptoms similar to this. It also crossed his mind that perhaps Teddi was more upset by her separation from Kim than anyone had imagined, and that the emotional trauma had triggered this physical reaction.

Gary told his daughter to try and calm down. "Just relax," he said. The urgency and fear in his voice did not go unnoticed by his son and wife. Gary tried to hold onto Teddi's arm but it jerked violently out of his hand, as if it had a life of its own.

"Call an ambulance," Sheri urged.

"I can't until I know what's wrong," he shot back.

Sheri demurred. "I don't know," she said, shaking her head. "But I think you ought to call one."

Sheri was afraid that some sort of paralysis was setting in and that Teddi's lungs would collapse. She called her pediatrician for advice. The doctor recommended that Teddi be brought by ambulance to Strong Memorial Hospital at once.

They were not prepared for the fact that the ambulance would take nearly forty-five minutes to arrive. The Mervis home in suburban Pittsford was only about seven miles from Rochester, where the hospital was, but the spring explosion of new growth had blocked the street sign. The ambulance couldn't find the house, and the Mervises tried to remain calm—for Teddi's sake—until it finally arrived about ten o'clock.

Gary and Sheri followed the ambulance as it stormed its way to the hospital. They could see Teddi vomiting. Her mother knew that Teddi hadn't vomited since she was about a year old, and that she would be frightened. Gary still kept thinking the cause of Teddi's problem was petit mal. As they turned into the hospital parking lot, he mentioned this to his wife. Sheri shrugged, and the scene flashed before her of Teddi having a seizure in school, and being embarrassed, and having her classmates reject her.

Several people, including nurses, the attending physician and other personnel, hovered around Teddi. The seizure activity worsened. Teddi was still vomiting. Her arm still shook violently, and it was discovered that she had no use of her left hand. The left side of Teddi's face was also twitching erratically; her mouth moving up and down silently, like a puppet's jaw.

The Mervises watched the feverish activity from its fringe. They took comfort in the arrival of the pediatrician that Sheri had called.

Though what was happening to her, and around her, was overwhelming, Teddi nevertheless struggled to maintain her composure. She had a strong will for a child so small. The hospital's official admission chart documented her response to standard orientation questions: "I am at Strong Memorial Hospital. The President is Carter. This is Thursday."

It was now just a little after midnight and Gary went to a phone to call his younger brother, Bob. He told Bob about what was happening, and asked if he minded picking up Tod and have the boy stay with him that night. Bob said of course he wouldn't mind. Gary promised to call him sometime later in the morning.

Gary then called Irene Matichyn. He told her what was going on and asked to speak to Kim. Kim, who had been asleep, came to the phone.

"This is daddy, honey," Gary said. "Teddi's pretty sick. Your mommy and I are here at Strong Memorial Hospital. What I wanted to know—did anything happen to Teddi today? Did she fall?" He paused. "Please tell me the truth, honey, did you push her or anything like that?"

Kim assured him that nothing like that happened. They talked some more and after saying good night, Kim sat down next to her friend Chrissy and began to cry. They both were soon crying, believing that if they hadn't left Teddi behind that day none of this would have happened.

Chrissy's mother, Irene, tossed and turned the remainder of the night. She kept going over the scene in her mind, Teddi standing in the garage alone, crying. She thought nobody wanted her, Irene repeated to herself. "We should have never caused her to feel so rejected."

Tod, Teddi's older brother, the more mischievous of the Mervis children, would also have a difficult time sleeping that night. Before bed he asked his uncle: "She's going to be okay, isn't she?" His uncle tried to reassure him.

Gary also placed a call to his friend Skip DeBiase. Though it was late, he knew that Skip and his wife Cheryl would want to be told. "Skip"—short for Salvatore—was president of Mohawk Printing Company where Gary worked. The couple were close friends of the Mervises.

Skip told Gary not to think the worst, that almost anything may have triggered the seizures. Gary agreed to stay calm and wait it out. He told Skip he'd call him later the following day.

Meanwhile, Teddi had been given Phenobarbital and Decadron. The twitching subsided but did not stop completely. A decision was made to keep Teddi there overnight for observation.

As she was being wheeled to the pediatric unit, the resident physician walking with them decided to take a detour. Why not take an X-ray of Teddi's head to see if they could find anything that may have caused the seizure? The X-ray was taken, nothing was found, and grins broke out all around.

It was dark and other children were asleep in the large room where Teddi was taken. She was exhausted at this point. "What time is it?" she asked her father. Her voice was but a whisper from the large bed in the large room.

Gary looked at his watch. "It's almost 2:30 in the morning," he told her.

Displaying some of the same matter-of-factness and honesty evident in her mother, Teddi's response was: "Oh, that's way past my bed time. I have to go to bed now."

Gary turned to his wife. "Maybe you better stay with her."

Sheri didn't like the idea. "Why me?" she wanted to know.

Gary was abrupt. "I can't stay in a hospital. I hate hospitals. I've never been in a hospital. And I never plan on being in one!"

Sheri maintained her control, even though she was angry. "I'm not particularly fond of them either," she answered.

They realized they were both tired and decided to go home together, get a good night's rest, and return to the hospital early the next morning. After all, the seizure activity had all but stopped now and Teddi began to look like she always did. The doctor told them that the medication would make her sleep until late the next morning.

Sheri kissed her daughter good night. They whispered back to each other "I love you." Then Gary kissed her. Before leaving he turned the radio on so that Teddi would have some soft music; he thought it might make her feel as though she were not alone.

The drive home was a relaxed one. Everything seemed to be in control. The X-ray didn't turn up anything. For all they knew a fall, or even something as minor as an allergic reaction to cats, may have triggered the seizures. The couple felt confident and slept soundly that first night.

2

The First Day

Early the next morning, the Mervises returned to the hospital. Gary drove this time and instead of going in, he decided to head for a downtown department store. He remembered Teddi talking about a special teddy bear in the store window and he wanted to get it for her now. He dropped off Sheri and went ahead.

Sheri walked directly to Teddi's room on the fourth floor of the hospital, the Pediatrics Unit. She paused in the doorway of Teddi's room and immediately saw an "iron lung," widely used in the days of polio. This one was small enough to hold a child. Sheri put her hand to her mouth to stop the emotion rising up inside her. 'Teddi's lung *did* collapse,' she thought to herself.

She turned. The night before there had been only a skeleton crew on duty, but now there was a full complement of nurses and a lot of activity. She could feel herself beginning to panic. She walked unsteadily toward the nurse's station.

"Did Teddi stop breathing?", she asked, point blank. The nurse was doing paperwork and now looked up.

"Who's Teddi?", the nurse asked.

"She's my daughter," Sheri answered. Though she had made the claim many times in the past, at no time were the words more painful to say than now. It was as if Sheri were not only laying a claim to her name but her life.

The nurse looked through some papers. "I'm sorry," she said, "but we don't have a Teddi here."

Sheri then motioned to Teddi's room of the night before. She thought maybe Teddi was in the thing that looked like an iron lung.

"Oh, no," the nurse answered. "His name is Johnny—Johnny's in that."

Sheri tried to hold back her tears. "Well, then where's Teddi?" And then she remembered, "Oh, try Elizabeth. Elizabeth Mervis. It's under that name."

The nurse again looked through her papers. She shook her head. "There's no Elizabeth Mervis here, either," she said.

"Does that mean that Teddi died during the night?" Sheri asked, surprised by her own words.

The nurse turned ashen, rose, and told Sheri to wait. The nurse then talked with others on the floor. A second nurse came over to where Sheri was standing. "Oh, I think I recall they put her in a private room next to the one she was in last night." The nurse pointed. "Over there," she said.

Sheri began walking to the room where the nurse had pointed. She and Gary had requested a private room the night before. She just wished somebody had told her from the start, saving her from all the aggravation and tense moments.

But when Sheri got to the room, it was empty. Another nurse came over to Sheri and said she thought they sent Teddi upstairs for some tests. Back at the nurse's station they placed a phone call upstairs but no one there had heard of a Teddi, or an Elizabeth, Mervis.

One of the nurses located Teddi's admission papers. Teddi had been exposed to chicken pox recently, and early that morning it was decided to move Teddi to the adult neurological unit to prevent possible contamination of other children on the floor.

Sheri went to Teddi's room on the sixth floor and was now shocked to see her daughter asleep beneath a plastic oxygen tent.

"Does she need that?", Sheri asked the nurse.

The nurse shrugged. "We thought she might need it," she answered. Minutes later the oxygen tent was removed.

Sheri sat beside her daughter. She gently rubbed Teddi's arm. Her daughter's face, normally pink, now looked pale; there were also dark shadows around her eyes. Teddi's hair, thick and curly, was matted in the back. Tears welled up inside of Sheri in reaction to how her daughter looked—and at the madness of the morning. Sheri disciplined her heart and didn't cry.

As soon as Teddi awakened she began vomiting. Her left side was nearly paralyzed, and because she was on medication, she was unable to move and began to choke. Sheri desperately tried to turn her over but the limp body was too heavy. She screamed for a nurse. The nurse who came told Sheri, matter-of-factly, "Oh, you have to tip her on her side like this."

Teddi was taken downstairs for a CT scan. Often referred to as a "cat" scan, the patient is positioned head first on a table which passes slowly through what looks like a giant, white-enameled doughnut. The scan provides pictures at one-inch intervals in an 180° arc. Painless, with no after effects, the entire process for the area of the brain takes about a half hour.

Yet Teddi nevertheless had to take the test alone in the brightly lit room. The heavy leaded doors were closed tight, and doctors observed the procedure from an adjacent room. Test results showed that there was scattered swelling on the right side of the brain.

Dr. Curtis N. Nelson stopped by Teddi's room after the test results became known. Handsome, athletic-looking, careful in the words he gave to patients and their families, Nelson introduced himself to the Mervises, including Teddi. He said he was a neurosurgeon. Sheri took an immediate liking to him. Her English heritage and mannerisms, her reserved style, coincided with Nelson's calm, almost emotionless, demeanor. Gary, on the other hand, was initially more uncomfortable with the doctor when they met a few days later. Dr. Nelson told Sheri that the couple probably wouldn't be in need of his services. He had examined Teddi and thought the child was progressing normally.

In the hospital chart for the day Dr. Nelson wrote that the CT scan was "not very suggestive of a tumor, though this is possible." He also noted that Teddi was "drowsy but wakens and gives name as 'Liz.' "

At that point, usually only her family, close relatives, and friends called her "Teddi." The name on her birth certificate was Elizabeth, named after Gary's mother, who had died suddenly when Sheri was pregnant with the girl. Gary had wanted to name her "Elizabeth," but Sheri, hoping for a boy, wanted the name "Ted." When the child was born she looked like a little teddy bear, Sheri thought. She was soft, pudgy, with furry crop of hair on her head, and so Sheri nicknamed her "Teddi"—changing the spelling to make it feminine and the name stuck.

Later that first day in the hospital, Teddi was given an Electroencephalogram, or more commonly known as an EEG. The test records brain wave activity on a moving sheet of graph paper and indicates whether the brain is functioning abnormally.

Teddi was tired, and Gary, after presenting her with a new teddy bear, was aware of how anxious she was becoming. While the medical personnel busily set up their equipment to conduct the EEG and prepared the two dozen electrodes to be attached to Teddi's head, Gary asked his daughter to whistle for him. That made Teddi laugh. Then Gary started laughing. Teddi, ever obedient, began to whistle. Gary was asked to leave.

Teddi's nurse noted in her report for that full day of activities that Teddi seemed lethargic, though arousable, through verbal stimulation. Teddi had vomited around 5:00 P.M. that day. At around 7:00 P.M., noted the nurse, Teddi was alert, talkative, and better oriented.

That evening, Gary's brother, Bob, Skip and Cheryl DeBiase, and a few other close friends and relatives arrived. Most thought Teddi didn't look bad at all. Most thought, like Gary, that Teddi had acquired some form of epilepsy but that with modern drugs, and other treatment, it could be controlled and Teddi would have a normal life. The Mervises expressed their concern that the medical staff was looking for problems that weren't really there. Gary thought the CT scan was going too far.

Irene Matichyn arrived late. When she saw Teddi, she sensed that something was deeply wrong. Skip, seeing her reaction, took her arm. Irene caught herself and didn't say anything, not even to Skip later, but she thought something in Teddi's eyes had changed, that something was different. Again she played over that scene in the driveway when she had come for her own daughter, and Kim, leaving Teddi crying and alone.

3

The Ante Goes Up

A second brain scan was done the following morning. Teddi was given radioisotopes this time. Radioisotopes are a non-radioactive chemical that allows the scanner to locate any abnormality in the brain without harming normal tissue or causing pain to the patient. Teddi was asked to change positions several times during the test so that views could be taken from front, back, and the side.

The brain scan was unofficially reported as normal and Dr. Nelson proposed a wait-and-see attitude. If the swelling in Teddi's head went down and her overall condition kept improving, maybe she could go home. In any case, he suggested that further testing be deferred for a few days.

No overt seizure activity was reported on that day, though it was clear that Teddi's left side was weak. Her grasp on that side was less than firm, and she had trouble walking. She also complained of numbness in her left hand and on the left side of her face. The nurse also thought she was moodier, noting in her chart that Teddi seemed to be "emotionally depressed."

An accident occurred early the following morning. The orderly who brought Teddi breakfast forgot to put the siderails up on her bed. Teddi fell from the bed and struck her head. A pediatrician was called to examine her but found no other damage than the bruise which was developing. But when Gary and Sheri Mervis arrived they were furious about what had happened.

A repeat CT scan was done that day. Dr. Nelson came to the room afterward. Trying not to over- or under-estimate the situation, he said the scan now definitely showed something. He wasn't sure, as yet, what it was. One thing he said it could be was an aneurism, explaining that it was a sac which formed on the wall of an artery as a result of disease or injury. Sheri winced, thinking of Teddi's fall earlier that morning. The doctor went on to say that the scan may be turning up something caused by the seizure activity itself. He also added it could be a tumor.

Sheri jumped. She wanted to know if it was cancerous or not.

"It's in the light gray area," Dr. Nelson told her, pointing it out to her on the scan. "That would indicate to me that it is not cancerous."

Sheri couldn't let go of her fear. "Are you sure?" she asked.

Nelson repeated that his experience with tumors taught him that if they were found in the light gray areas they were generally not cancerous.

Sheri asked a third time. "Did you say *not* cancer?" And then she spelled out the word "not."

He nodded. "That's right," he said.

Sheri did not fear tumors, if they weren't cancerous. She felt relieved now. In her childhood she had had a tumor removed from her leg. The doctor had made a slit, popped it out, and snipped it off. But when Gary heard that there might be a tumor growing inside his daughter's head, an old fear surged within him.

Though never an avid reader, Gary did remember a book that had a tremendous impact upon him as a youngster, a book he read cover to cover despite its sad tale. It was John Gunther's *Death Be Not Proud*, the author's personal account of the death of his son as a result of a malignant brain tumor. The book had haunted Gary all of his life.

A shift was now occurring in the response of the Mervises to developments with respect to Teddi. Sheri, upon hearing that the tumor was in all probability not cancerous, returned to Teddi's bedside. She would leave the medical and other details to Gary and instead concentrate her efforts on comforting Teddi.

Dr. Nelson suggested to Gary that they do a cerebral angiogram. The swelling in Teddi's brain had not diminished and he wanted to find out why. But the ante was raised and the stakes were getting higher. A cerebral angiogram contained inherent dangers. There was a consent form to sign.

The form was written in the first person, and so Gary would be signing for his daughter. It stated:

> . . . using sterile technique and local anesthesia (novacaine) a needle will be placed in my groin, a flexible tube passed through the needle, and the tubing advanced into vessels going to head and neck; then dye will be injected and pictures taken with x-ray.

The form also explained some of the details of the procedure and then went on to cite the potential risks involved: stroke, bleeding, clot formation, infection, respiratory complication, and reaction to the anesthesia.

Gary couldn't bring himself to sign the form. He talked it over with his wife and both agreed they needed some time to think it over. Though both never said it out loud, each hoped that by postponing a decision they could buy a little time for Teddi. Maybe she would get better. Maybe she could go home and all the tests would stop.

It wasn't a vain hope. On the surface at least, Teddi was definitely looking better. The Phenobarbital was controlling the seizure activity. Teddi was gaining increasing use of her left hand and was generally becoming more active. Teddi herself kept asking why she couldn't go home.

Later that evening two doctors entered the room. One, the Mervises later recalled, was to die a few months later in the crash of a DC–10 out of Chicago. The accident became an important lesson to the Mervises in terms of the value of each moment of each day, even for the healthy and strong.

The doctors had come with the intention of convincing the Mervises that signing the consent form for the cerebral angiogram was the right thing to do.

After hearing them out, Gary shook his head. "It's pretty powerful stuff to be asked to make a decision for someone else based upon so little information . . ." He paused. His voice faltered, just for an instant, but it did not go unnoticed. Then Gary added: " . . . especially someone so precious to you."

One of the doctors spoke up. "Well, you know, Mr. Mervis," he said, "we're talking about something that's potentially very serious. If the neurosurgeon has to operate, he needs to know where the blood supply is— where the vessels are. The only way he can know that is with the results from an angiogram."

Gary wavered. The other doctor intervened. "We're talking about your daughter's life, Mr. Mervis," he said, his voice rising. "The possibility of surgery is increasing every day. If it's an aneurism or a tumor then it will require surgery to correct."

Gary wanted to know the details of the doctor's argument.

The doctor explained that if it was aneurism, they would operate and try to repair the blood vessel. If it was a tumor, on the other hand, they would try to take it out. "You must understand," said the doctor, "that the neurosurgeon is not able to do anything unless he has those results."

The next morning Teddi was wheeled into a large room lined with wooden cabinets containing medicine and angiogram testing materials. Placed on her back, Teddi was given a local anesthetic. A liquid called dye (though it is clear) was to run through a catheter but the effort to put the catheter in Teddi's artery, near her groin, failed. After several more time-consuming tries, the staff tried the artery on the opposite side of Teddi's groin. These efforts also failed.

Meanwhile, the local anesthesia was wearing off, and Teddi was getting restless. It was imperative that Teddi be able to lie perfectly still because the angiogram requires the catheter to be threaded through Teddi's system of arteries until it is able to reach the brain. The radiologist's job was to guide the catheter through this network of blood vessels through the use of a fluroscope, which provided a picture of the catheter's movement. The fluroscope was like a small TV and hung just above the table.

Because the anesthesia was wearing off, the doctors thought they would postpone the test until the following morning. The danger was that a restless Teddi could cause the catheter to pierce or otherwise bruise a blood vessel, causing a clot, which could result in death.

Gary and Sheri were waiting impatiently for news from the doctor. The procedure, they had been told, could take anywhere from one to four hours. Teddi had been in the room for four hours and now all three were told they had to go through it all again the following morning.

On the fifth day of Teddi's stay in the hospital, April 24, 1979, the doctor's performed the angiogram, this time applying general anesthesia. They were successful in inserting the catheter this time and the angiogram was completed. Attempts were made to lift Teddi from her anesthesia at about 12:15 P.M. At about 2:30 that afternoon, she was alert, complaining she was hungry. She took short naps. Her condition after the second angiogram attempt was described as stable but uncomfortable.

She was looking even more alert and aware by suppertime. Gary mentioned to the nurse he believed the muscle tone in Teddi's face had improved. He also told the nurse that she was walking more that day. Her grasp was better, and her smile, he thought, looked almost normal again. The nurse reported these comments and observed that Teddi seemed increasingly worried about what was happening to her.

Dr. Nelson brought the results of the angiogram to Teddi's room that night. The angiogram showed a mass in the brain. He favored a craniotomy and biopsy.

Gary reacted in anger, masking his pain and shock. "Why weren't there any signs?" he wanted to know. "Why didn't we notice it? Why weren't there any problems before Teddi had that first seizure?"

Nelson interrupted, trying to comfort this father whose eyes now reddened. It was the doctor's strong belief that the tumor was in a place that didn't control anything—that wouldn't affect Teddi physically or psychologically.

It was now Gary's turn to interrupt. "Tumor? Did you say tumor?"

Nelson nodded. "Yes. It appears to be a low-grade tumor. But it *is* operable."

The doctor went on to explain that he believed the tumor to be a low-grade astrocytoma tumor because the astrocytoma doesn't normally receive a lot of blood. This deficiency of blood, Nelson thought, might explain why it didn't show up on the CT scan, which is about ninety-eight percent accurate in diagnosing brain tumors. The good news, he told the Mervises, is that the astrocytoma tumor, when found in children, is not generally cancerous. He said that type of tumor most often showed up in older people.

Gary shook his head, repeating the same phrase again and again. "I want you to be very aggressive and get it all out," he told the doctor.

Nelson responded with the words: "Once you two get over the fact that what she has is a tumor—get used to that, then everything else will be all right."

Nelson explained the risks, complications, and alternatives to the Mervises, including Teddi. He wanted to schedule surgery for the 27th, two days from then, and the three members of the Mervis family agreed to go ahead with the operation.

Nelson left and the adult Mervises tried to put a positive spin on these new developments. They went over the basic facts for Teddi's benefit, and their own: it was a low-grade tumor; that type of tumor was generally not cancerous; and it was in an area that wasn't considered dangerous.

There were other things to consider as well. Dr. Nelson had a great reputation as a surgeon. Though they knew the waiting and wondering would be hard, they believed that once the surgery was over and Teddi recuperated, they could all forget about this unspeakable moment in their lives and go back to being a family with normal problems and challenges.

4

A World Comes Apart

The new morning brought more anxiety and apprehension, as Gary reviewed the latest consent form that he would have to sign. He didn't like it. Its contents, the risks and complications, were even more serious than the angiogram. The consent form this time contained, as a possible risk, the word "death."

A nurse whose nickname was "Charlie" had befriended Teddi. She sometimes even came in to see the child on her day off. Now she tried to comfort Teddi who was extremely upset because her head was going to have to be completely shaved for surgery.

"Why can't this have happened to me when I was smaller and didn't know anything about it?", she complained. "I'm going to look awful without my hair. I wish I could die rather than have no hair."

Charlie read Teddi a book about surgery, supplied by the pediatric unit. Teddi cried at certain points. She talked about her fears regarding the operation. She said she was afraid of surgery, and also of dying.

Nurse Anne Cameron came down from the pediatric unit to greet Teddi and to escort her on a tour of her unit. Young, gentle in her ways, and a good nurse, Anne and Teddi quickly became friends. Their tour together, it seemed, lightened Teddi's sadness some.

Nothing unusual marked Teddi's preparation for surgery. Routine blood and urine tests were conducted; there was a meeting with the anesthesiologist who conducted a pre-operative evaluation, which included selection of the proper anesthesia. Teddi was allowed a light supper the night before surgery, and then would have to fast until the operation was over.

Bob Mervis, Skip and Cheryl DeBiase, Irene, and a few other close friends and relatives stopped by the night before the operation to comfort the Mervises and to wish Teddi good luck. They all said they would return the following day except Irene. She had a demanding workload to take care of.

She made Sheri promise, instead, to call her once Teddi was out of surgery. Irene would come then.

It was quiet in the room now.

"How soon can I go home?" Teddi asked.

"We'll see, honey," said her mother, glancing quickly over at Gary. "The operation will hurt some afterwards," Sheri said, "but not before that. But it's nothing you can't tolerate, honey."

Gary explained to her again that she had a tumor in her head, and why they had to take it out. Teddi wanted her dad to explain what a tumor was like. And Gary told her once again that it was kind of like a mass of things—of cells—that had grown into a ball. He told her to just make it through the operation, and after that, whatever she wanted, he would try to get for her.

Sheri and Gary assured their daughter that they would be there the following morning before she went into surgery. Teddi eventually fell asleep, and her parents kissed her, each alone with their own thoughts and prayers.

As they were leaving, the new resident physician came in to introduce herself. She said she would be participating in the operation. The Mervises wanted to know if it were possible for her to leave the operating room at any point and tell them how Teddi was doing. She assured them that at about half-way through the surgery she'd be able to leave momentarily. The Mervises felt even better as they headed for home.

Early the next morning, Teddi was further "prepped" for the craniotomy, including premedication to help relax her. Teddi's parents arrived, as did her Uncle Bob, the nurse named "Charlie," and a few others. They all walked with her as she was wheeled, on a long table, to the operating room.

Her parents were the last to say good-bye. Gary kissed his daughter. "Don't worry, honey," he said. "Everything will be all right." Sheri couldn't speak. She squeezed Teddi's hand instead. Just before Teddi entered the operating room she asked "Charlie" if it was all right to let Teddietta, her bear, stay with her. Charlie told her it would be all right.

The main area where the Mervises had to wait was busy with human traffic. The electronically operated doors dominated the lobby, and seemed to open and close thousands of times during the seven hours they were to wait. Strangers rushed by, or paused to ask directions of the receptionist. They looked for a familiar face. They also seemed to hold hands more than they did outside.

Not long after Teddi went into surgery, a nurse came from the operating room and gave Teddietta, the bear, to Sheri. Sheri spent some of the long wait bandaging Teddietta's head so that it would look like Teddi's, after the operation. Maybe Teddi wouldn't feel so different and alone afterward. Gary talked with well-wishers who had come by during the day. He spent time with Skip, who kept trying to reassure Gary that everything would be all right.

The sounds of a drill and saw dominated the initial activity in the operating room. Dr. Nelson first made a rectangular incision on the cleanly shaved scalp on the middle right of Teddi's head. Four holes, each just a little smaller than a dime, were then drilled into Teddi's skull. The holes were connected with a saw cut and the window of bone was removed.

A leathery membrane prevented Dr. Nelson from having a clear view of Teddi's brain. He proceeded slowly, looking for signs of the tumor. Then he cut into the membrane and could feel his own heart sink.

To his surprise, and dismay, Teddi's tumor had invaded the surface of the brain. Multiple implants were also visible. He now cut down into the tumor itself. It was rubbery. He took a piece from the tumor's surface and sent it out for a frozen section. This would give him a preliminary reading as to the tumor's true nature.

Dr. Nelson continued to explore the tumor. He found it had grown in, and among, the brain tissue. The tumor had not only altered the brain's consistency, it presented dangerously few clear borders marking it from the brain itself. It had grown wildly, looking like the tentacles of an octopus, strangling parts of the brain and entangling itself elsewhere. Getting the entire tumor out would be impossible.

Based upon what he saw, and the returned biopsy report, Nelson the man would now dominate Nelson the doctor. Curtis Nelson decided that the location and interlocking nature of Teddi's tumor meant that if he were to cut into the brain, the child might suffer personality changes and in all likelihood would end up paralyzed on her left side. Removing as much of the tumor as he could may not cure the child, but it might diminish her capacity to have a normal experience in the time she had left.

Nelson put back the window of bone and unfolded the patch of scalp over it. He closed the incision. It was perfunctory work, and his thoughts turned to what he would say to the Mervises. He knew that the most difficult part of his day was still ahead of him.

The Mervises were extremely agitated at this point. Sheri fidgeted with Teddietta while she sat in one of the large, brown hospital chairs. Gary paced, then stopped in front of Skip. "We'll have her out dancing tonight," Skip joked, trying to cheer Gary up. Bob Mervis sat in a chair watching.

One by one they saw Dr. Nelson, and a resident physician, walking toward them. Cheryl DeBiase remembers seeing a smile on Dr. Nelson's face and was sure he was going to say that everything was all right. Skip, her husband, felt himself grow cold, and tried to slip into the background. Bob Mervis could never remember the moment.

"We'd like to talk with you," Nelson said, motioning the Mervises toward the surgical waiting area—a more private part of the lobby. Sheri's knees buckled. Gary felt a terrible moan rising up inside him. They walked as if in a trance, oblivious to all sounds and movements and faces around them.

Sheri sat down in a chair near the window; Gary standing beside her. Not far from them was a sculpture by Achille Forgione. One of the figures in the sculpture played a mandolin, the other a flute. Carved in stone were the words:

> . . . Gently they go, the beautiful
>   the tender, the kind;
> Quietly they go, the intelligent
>   the witty, the brave. . . .

Dr. Nelson's words drifted in and out of the trance the Mervises found themselves in. He seemed rattled. "I was so surprised when I opened her up and saw the cancer," he said. "I was so surprised I couldn't believe it."

He told them Teddi's condition was extremely bad, that the biopsy taken during surgery revealed that the tumor was malignant. He told them what he had found, that the tumor was in a section of the brain that was critical to Teddi's life, that he did not try to take very much of it out. As bad as that was, he went on to say that the immediate concern was whether or not Teddi would survive the surgery itself.

Nelson continued, telling the Mervises that they were going to have to begin exploring forms of treatment other than surgery to combat the tumor. He explained some of the alternatives, commented upon their feasibility and affects, and offered his opinion. But the Mervises had stopped hearing.

They had been waiting for seven hours for Teddi to come out of surgery, to just get through that part of it. They had come to believe that surgery was the last step—not the first, in Teddi's ordeal. Never had they contemplated Teddi's death, either now or in the forseeable future.

Nelson and the resident physician left the Mervises. Sheri's mother then went to her, alone, and then she returned to tell the others what had happened. Cheryl DeBiase slipped her arm around Sheri. She remembers Sheri being tense, almost stern, except for the slow tears that began to fall down her face. They hugged each other, the women present, squeezing the bandaged Teddietta close to Sheri's heart.

As Gary turned, Skip could see that Gary's eyes were red. He got closer and saw tears beginning to stream down Gary's face. As their arms met, Skip felt Gary go limp. He held him. "Come," he said, "walk with me."

As they passed by the electronic doors to the outside, Gary began to cry. "Why? Why my baby?" he was crying. "Why Teddi?"

Skip still wasn't sure what exactly had happened but it no longer seemed to matter. He made himself stop crying. His friend needed him. He could feel sorry for himself later.

Skip kept saying things to try and reassure Gary, who was still crying, and asking why. He didn't remember what he said but that didn't seem to matter either, it was almost as if the sounds the words made, the comfort of the sound, mattered more than the words themselves.

"Gary," he told his friend, "whatever it is it's going to work out. And it might look bad right now but they're coming up with things all the time. She's going to be responsive to treatments." He kept talking and all the while knew Gary wasn't listening to a single word.

Suddenly, after about twenty minutes, Gary caught hold of himself. "Where's Sheri?" he asked Skip.

Skip took the remark as a sign that Gary had pulled himself back together and was ready to go back inside. He took Gary's arm, and walked toward the hospital door.

It was like a slow motion scene in the movies. Those beside Sheri began to slowly leave her side just as Gary, overwhelmed by the sorrow in his heart, had to see the same sorrow in his wife's eyes. There was never a harder moment in all the time to follow than this one.

At that very moment Irene came bouncing through the main lobby, looking for Sheri. She had been worried, then angry, that Sheri hadn't called her at work as she promised. "Damn it!" she had remembered saying, "I'm one of her closest friends and she hasn't even called."

Irene stopped suddenly. She saw Skip and Cheryl both crying. She began to shake, to sob. She knew it was going to be bad; deep in her heart she had known it was going to be bad.

She and Skip met each other half way, Irene collapsing in his arms. "It isn't good," Skip whispered to her. "They're worried she might not even make it through the day."

"Where are Sheri and Gary?" she asked, weeping heavily now.

"Be strong," Skip answered. "They need you to be strong."

Irene found Gary and could see he was devastated. Though they had worked together for five years, sometimes ten hours a day, they had never hugged each other. They did now.

Sheri had slipped away from the others and was now trying to gain entry into the recovery room. A nurse stood in the doorway, forbidding entrance. Only medical personnel could go in.

Sheri grew suspicious. First they told her it wasn't cancer, and now it was. Then they said they were going to take the entire tumor out but they hadn't. Was Teddi dead? Is that why they didn't want her to go in? She let out a painful cry.

Sheri was allowed to go in but only for a moment. She could see that Teddi was breathing. Though her eyes were bleary from the tears, she managed to put the bandaged Teddietta next to the bandaged Teddi.

Gary had also left the others now. He found Dr. Nelson talking to another doctor and interrupted. He began to ask every question that was rushing through his mind.

Nelson, aware there was still a great deal about the tumor he needed to know, couldn't be of much help professionally. "Well, Mr. Mervis," he said, "I've got to be careful how I talk to you."

Gary interpreted Nelson's hesitation as being that of a man afraid. He exploded. "Forget about me suing you or anything like that!" he shouted. "I've got two other kids at home! I've got to go back and tell them what the hell is happening!" And then the words came out, the words Gary himself dreaded putting in the air. "What are we talking about, Doctor? Christmas? Is she going to be alive by Christmas?"

"I don't know," Nelson answered. All he could tell Gary, he said, was that the next twenty-four to forty-eight hours were going to be critical. She needed to make it through recovery without infections or other serious complications.

Gary wasn't satisfied. "I'm not going to let you off the hook," he told Nelson. "It's not my nature. You're Teddi's doctor now and you're going to stay with us until the end."

5

Wrestling with the Devil

Nearly three hours after the operation the elevator doors opened and Teddi was wheeled out on a bed. Her head was bandaged, and iodine dripped from beneath the white gauze. Her face looked almost bruised, ashen and blue with a tinge of green. The bandaged Teddietta lay beside her.

Sheri touched Teddi's face and found it freezing cold. "They lied to me," she muttered, too soft for the others to hear. "They lied to me. She's going to die right now. She's gone."

An orderly wheeled the bed slowly down the corridor, her parents following. Sheri's mother, Bob, Skip, Cheryl, Irene, and a few others also walked behind. They held hands randomly, each alone with their thoughts. Heads shook in disbelief and grief.

Once Teddi entered the intensive care unit, the medical staff hurriedly went to work. First they hooked her up to a heart monitor. Small, like a television set, three wires connected it to the body with a sticky substance. The apparatus is so sensitive that if the patient moved suddenly, a shrill, persistent alarm sounded.

Two I.V.s from a pressure pump measured the amount of fluid entering Teddi's body. It was necessary because any error in measurement after surgery could be fatal. The machine was also capable of alerting the staff if air entered the tube or if the fluid was going into the skin rather than a vein. In terms of these problems, and others, a different kind of alarm was sounded.

A long tube extended from another bottle, in through Teddi's nose, and ending in her stomach. From it, a greenish-yellow fluid slowly dripped from Teddi's stomach back into the bottle. This was to drain her stomach so she wouldn't vomit. Over Teddi's head, on a shelf, was a black bag used when breathing stopped. Each of the six beds in the pediatric intensive care unit had a similar setup. The room was either noisy or quiet. That afternoon it was very noisy.

Gary watched, eyes reddened, as Skip poked at Teddi's cheek.

She opened one eye, a smile starting in the corner of her mouth.

"Don't you bat those eyelashes at me," he kidded.

Almost immediately Teddi drifted back into sleep.

Skip looked up at Gary. "It can't be," he said, shaking his head. He left the room. He felt himself short circuiting and left the hospital to walk in the parking lot alone.

Teddi spent a restless first night after surgery. There was almost constant activity in the room. Every hour for the first ten hours, her heart-rate, respirations and blood pressure were checked. Neuro checks were also done nearly every hour. Their purpose was to test whether her brain was functioning normally. Nearly every hour a nurse opened Teddi's eyelids and looked in with a flashlight to see if her pupils restricted as they should have.

Teddi was also awakened each hour and asked her name, how old she was, where she lived, and if she knew where she was. Despite the apparent absurdity of waking somebody so gravely ill, the procedure was vital: failure to respond properly was a first sign of increased pressure on the brain. The condition was considered critical.

The Mervises, too, spent a restless night. Sheri went over the past, all that led to that moment. She thought about the future, the slow undoing of all their lives, the slow breaking of her heart. She prayed for courage, and also, if need be, for mercy.

Gary was angry at God. Why would God want to take a child? he wondered. His child? His Teddi? Why wasn't a crook or rapist or murderer chosen instead of his baby? He wondered why God hadn't picked him instead.

What made it hard was that Teddi was such a good person, thoughtful of others, cheerful and kind. Moreover, important to Gary, she carried his mother's name. Gary's mother was central to his life. She had encouraged him through all his difficult years of raising a family, going to school, becoming his own person.

His mother had died relatively young, at the age of fifty-one, choking to death on the floor of a restaurant while Gary, Bob, and Sheri—pregnant with Teddi—frantically tried to revive her. Skip would note that whenever Gary talked about his mother, it was the only time he showed emotion. "Not a day goes by," he told Skip once, "that I don't think about my mother." He also told Skip that he didn't think anything as devastating would ever happen to him.

Unable to sleep, Gary went into the kitchen. He had a glass of water. He looked at the clock. It was three-thirty. Then he sat at the table. Sheri had fallen asleep by now; Tod and Kim were staying at the houses of others.

He wondered about his two other children, fast approaching adolescence. How would he tell them? How would it affect them? He wondered about his wife, his Sheri, and how she would hold up under the strain. Could their marriage endure the struggle and pain ahead?

His thoughts turned to his own life and career. Every decision in his control during the course of his political life had been carefully calculated to maximize his strengths and to bring him to the center of power. For eight years he made contacts, developed his skills, and built a reputation as one of the best campaign managers around. He was one of the youngest and best of a new breed of Republican politicos.

Gary wondered what would happen to all that now? Would the power brokers in Albany dismiss him now that there was something else on Gary's mind, something without parallel? Where would it all lead, he wondered, again and again.

Just a month before this development, he had taken a position offered to him by his friend Skip. Skip, president of Mohawk Printing, was his friend and would understand what he was going through. But how long could he lean on him? How well could Skip's business compete when a key team player had his heart elsewhere? Gary wondered if he'd be able to hang onto his job. Would developments affect his friendship with Skip? If he couldn't hold onto his job, then how would he support his family? Keep the house? Keep his self-respect?

Gary pushed himself away from the table. He looked out the window, staring into the darkness. He thought about Teddi again, remembered how her face looked after surgery, how bruised it was—the gauze, the iodine dripping down. He wondered how much time Teddi had left. Would the hospital be calling to tell him she was dead? Would he and Sheri arrive at the hospital that morning to find the room empty, the bed being readied for a new patient? Would anybody except God really know for sure how much time his daughter had left to live? Gary's anger returned now, but this time he wasn't sure who or what he was supposed to be mad at.

Then something began to change inside him. Those who know Gary Mervis know he's not the type of person to feel sorry for himself, at least not for long. Those who know him know he's not the type of person who likes being on the sidelines, or part of the crowd, or stuck in the audience.

Had Gary Mervis been born in a different part of town, or in a different city or even era, he might have become a winning football coach—the manager of a world-champion boxer. Instead, he chose to compete in politics, traditionally the place where dreams and self-interest, purpose and practicality nestle together under the same roof.

Though involved in politics for only seven years, he had already managed, or helped to manage, more than 150 state and local campaigns. Restless, even bored with the day-to-day functioning of government, Gary Mervis' passion was for the race itself. Though soft-spoken and even a little shy, inside he was a ferocious competitor who loved to win.

One thing Gary began to understand was that no matter how brief Teddi's life might be, he wasn't going to be on the sidelines any longer, leaving her fate to others. "I owe Teddi more than that," he said, in the empty house, startled by the words spoken out loud.

A new campaign began to take shape in his mind. This time it wasn't going to be politics, it was going to be for his daughter. He'd use what he had learned, lean on people he knew, and he wouldn't quit until he had his Teddi back on her feet. On the wall of his office at Mohawk Printing were Vince Lombardi's words—"Winning isn't everything, it's the only thing." Teddi would later tell one of her counselors: "My dad is not a quitter, and neither am I."

There was a relationship between politics—even war and cancer—long before Gary Mervis selected to join the fray. President Richard Nixon had proclaimed a "war against cancer" in 1973; doctors describe the disease as "the enemy." Medical textbooks talk about cancer as being an "army" of cells "invading" or "infiltrating" healthy parts of the body. These cells cross "borders" and "frontiers" without "provocation." An "aggressor," cancer had to be dealt with swiftly and aggressively, usually with a "surgical operation," like they had done in Vietnam. The struggle for the "hearts and minds" of the combatant and victim alike didn't get talked about much, as if failure belonged in another place.

The campaign Gary Mervis was to embark on was against a tiny cell in his daughter's head that had somehow gone berserk—dividing and subdividing, and dividing and subdividing over and over again until it outpaced the growth of healthy cells—"good" cells. The bad cell and its terrible offspring, now a mass inside of Teddi's head, is medically described as "malignant." The word also means "evil."

"Evil" pushed Gary's battle to a higher plane. People were afraid of cancer, afraid even of saying the word out loud, as if doing so would somehow awaken it, beckon it to one's own door.

Cancer seemed to mock America's faith in the infallibility of doctors and the ability of science and technology to defeat any foe. Cancer had become synonymous with death itself, sinister and mysterious, unpredictable in its coming, indiscriminate in the lives it claimed. It was a twentieth-century plague.

Gary Mervis was about to begin the toughest and most important campaign of his life. It would require everything he knew and all of his energy. He would need to learn all there was to know about the opposition, and recruit to his side the very best there was in the medical world. He would have to lean on others, and ask those he had helped to now help him.

The campaign Gary Mervis was about to wage was a campaign of the heart. Its goal was to save Teddi's life. And the competition was as small as a cell and as big as God.

6

Starting Over

Gary showered and dressed. He paced. He wandered about as dawn's first light filtered into the house. Around him was his life, what he had worked and sacrificed for, all he had built. He walked into the bedroom used by Teddi and Kim, which was empty now. He knew he was back to square one, that he and Sheri would have to struggle uphill again.

He and his wife had married young, just out of high school, and nobody—not even their parents—thought that their relationship would last. Gary had come from the city, from a working-class family who struggled and scraped, never owning a home. In contrast, Sheri's father came from the corporate world, her family owned a lovely suburban home.

After exchanging their marriage vows, Gary, a family man now, went to college full-time and worked full-time. In a typical day he would come home after work, talk to his wife briefly, look in on his kids, and then stay up late doing his homework. On weekends Gary hustled other jobs to bring in extra money for his growing family.

Finishing college, Gary had taken a job in New Jersey, commuting home to Rochester every other weekend. Then he began to work in Albany, as a chief legislative aide. Always, it was away from his family, his children. Ironically, he was to leave his job in Albany just a month before all this happened. He wanted to spend more time at home.

Because of school and work, Sheri assumed most of the responsibility for raising the children, and caring for household details. "She's an extraordinary woman," her next door neighbor, Betty Scobell would comment. "You could see her mowing the lawn in the morning, on a ladder fixing the gutters in the afternoon, and at night she would be looking absolutely radiant in an evening gown."

What Gary had done seemed absurd to him now. He had worn out his heart in order to make a decent living for his family and in the process had sacrificed his time with them. Now time would be the only priority.

Sheri listened as he talked, sitting on the bed. He told her of his desire to consult with the best doctors in the world and to search out what was being done by way of curing brain tumors in children. Sheri nodded, understanding her husband's driving love, and the nature of his heart.

Then they talked about other matters, practical matters. They had read about and seen stories on the news; in fact they knew personal examples of people who lost everything they owned because of the onset of catastrophic illness. Now with a sudden wrenching swiftness, like an oncoming tornado, their own lives had completed changed.

How much was in their savings account? How much would Blue Cross/ Blue Shield cover? They searched their insurance policies, talked of taking out a second mortgage on their home.

The fullness of the morning sun was upon them now. Outside, a dog was barking. Down the street a garage door opened. And Sheri and Gary agreed, just as the world was awakening, to spend whatever money it might take to save Teddi's life.

Gary then called his brother Bob to ask if they could meet at the library. Bob didn't hesitate. "Sure," he said.

The nights had been hard for Bob. Like everyone else close to Teddi, he thought the operation would be successful and everything would return to normal. But when he heard Teddi might die he had become deeply sad, even depressed. He was not only troubled for Teddi, but for his brother. Bob poured himself a second cup of coffee. As it did for Gary and the others, the past seemed to loom up, large, cutting, and in some ways comforting.

Though Gary had been the older brother, Bob felt he had been the one to take care of Gary. He remembered ironing his brother's clothes, sometimes cooking for him, and making him lunch. He thought his brother was almost helpless in such matters, and could never be self-sufficient. Yet he also admired his brother's capacity to motivate, organize and manage people.

Gary and Bob spent the day researching magazines, journals and newspapers. They looked for anything remotely related to Teddi's special type of tumor and the kinds of treatment available for such tumors. When they found something that looked useful, Gary, in his careful, neat handwriting, recorded it on a yellow legal pad.

Skip went to the hospital early that morning. He didn't knock at Teddi's door for fear of waking her. As he slipped silently inside, he found Sheri, sitting on the bed. He took the moment in.

Sheri was holding Teddietta. Teddi was awake and Sheri stroked her hand. She also occasionally stroked Teddietta. "God only knows," he thought, "where a mother would be at a time like this." In a way Skip was grateful that visitors were allowed in intensive care for only a few minutes.

Afterward, Skip went looking for Gary at the library. He was surprised at the look in Gary's eyes; different from the night before. Skip saw that the fight, and the hope, were back in Gary's eyes. A father himself, he knew if his child faced death he'd move heaven and hell to try and stop it.

"I've got to find out who to contact, Skipper," Gary said. "I've got to make sure Teddi will get the best care possible. I owe her that." He told Skip that he was going to do anything and everything possible to save his daughter's life. If he had to take her to the four corners of the globe, he'd do it. If he had to spend every dollar he had, and every minute he had to find a cure, then he'd do that, too. He said he wasn't going to have Teddi die only to have somebody say afterward: "Well, you know Gary, there is a guy in Taiwan you should have talked to. He might have helped." Gary Mervis was looking for gold and he wasn't going to leave a stone unturned. "A man possessed" was how Skip described him at this point. Skip joined the two brothers at the long wooden table looking up books, articles and magazines.

Bob Mervis would photocopy the longer pieces, the ones that weren't overly technical and seemed close to what they wanted. The stacks of collected material grew higher. The list of doctors and hospitals that might be of help grew longer. What started to bother them, however, was the accumulated evidence of what they were finding. There didn't seem to be much agreement as to the cause and cure of malignant tumors in children. Much of what they were reading was still experimental; others of it speculative.

Gary relieved Sheri at the hospital for part of that afternoon and evening. Teddi seemed to be doing well given the circumstances. Her right hand and grasp was stronger than that of her left hand, but she was able to move all her extremities now. She talked some, though her speech was somewhat halting.

An argument developed between Gary and one of the doctors. Skip had arrived but tried to stay in the background.

" . . . When can I get one of you guys to sign a form like the ones you make me sign?" Gary was saying, his voice rising. "When can I get you to do what you promise you'll do?"

"We're not God," the doctor answered coldly.

Skip couldn't restrain himself. He stepped forward. "Then why in hell do you act like you're God?" he asked.

The next morning the Mervises met with Teddi's pediatrician and Dr. Nelson, who had operated on Teddi. Gary told them both he was going to seek other opinions as to Teddi's diagnosis and potential treatments. "I have made a list of some of the best doctors in the world, and I plan on contacting them. I would like your fullest cooperation."

Nelson was uneasy. He wondered if the Mervises were going to go hospital shopping, desperate for a miracle cure that didn't exist. He had confidence in the personnel, technology, and care at Strong Memorial Hospital and told Gary he didn't think there was much point in looking elsewhere. "If you want a second opinion, Mr. Mervis," he said, "we can get one for you."

Gary shook his head. He told him he wanted to do that himself. He was going to personally send out Teddi's records, tests, and reports, and receive the results himself. He wanted the information to move swiftly, directly and with a minimal potential for error. He owed Teddi that, too.

The doctors tried to convince Gary that the people he wanted to contact were very prominent in the field and would in all likelihood be unavailable to him.

Gary listened, taking it all in, mulling over how he'd get them to listen. He knew he had done a lot of favors for people, some of whom owed their present jobs to him, and he could count on at least some of them for help. He could count on past political debts. He had helped a lot of people over the years, often sacrificing time with his own family. Now it would be his turn to ask. If he couldn't open the doors himself, he would try to get others to do it for him, even if it meant asking a state legislator or a United States Senator.

When the doctors finished, Gary gave them one line. "I don't want you people to take the next step in Teddi's care until I've had a chance to talk to these people."

Nelson told him not to wait long, that Teddi's survival may depend upon an early decision regarding treatment.

The Mervises walked in silence to the new wing of the hospital and took the elevator to Teddi's room. They were stunned by what they found. Teddi's face was swollen so much that her eyes were squeezed shut.

"Daddy, am I blind? I can't see, Daddy," Teddi was crying. She was sitting up in bed and reached out her arms toward the sound of their footsteps.

They calmed Teddi. Then Gary stormed from the room. He was stopping whomever he could find: "What the hell is going on? Can't somebody tell us what is going on so that little girl in there doesn't have to live in terror when she wakes up every morning?"

After that, at least one of the Mervises arrived early each morning and stayed late each night. They left only when Teddi was deep asleep, and the floor quiet, when they could reasonably be sure that nothing adverse was happening, or would happen, to Teddi. Even still, they phoned the hospital from home at night to check on her. The mother and father would be mother and father to their daughter at home—or in the hospital.

7

Looking for Miracles

The following morning, Gary placed a phone call to Kathleen Rose in Albany. Kathleen was Assemblyman James Nagle's administrative assistant and secretary, a person whom Gary had helped obtain her present job. Gary was Nagle's assistant in Rochester.

"Kathleen," Gary said. "How are you?"

"I'm fine," she answered. "I heard about things at your end and I'm sorry. Very, very sorry. Is there anything we can do?"

"Yes," said Gary. "I need your help."

"Name it," Kathleen said.

Gary smiled. This was one of those people he would have to lean on a great deal.

He went on to explain the essentials of what had happened, and said he needed her help in two major areas. First, he was seeking professional agreement as to Teddi's pathology report. "Pathology," in medical circles, was the attempt to understand the nature of a disease. In Teddi's case, Gary wanted to find out about the tumor. Was it a low-grade tumor? Slow growing? Was it highly malignant? How soon would it start to grow and expand again?

Determining the degree of malignancy would influence the course of Teddi's therapy, which would be the second search that Gary wanted to conduct. He wanted to find the latest and best cancer therapy and therapists available, no matter where he had to go, no matter what it might cost.

Kathleen Rose would be a key person in Gary's quest for information and advice. She was good at investigative research. She was dependable and persistent. She would make the phone calls, track down leads, suggest new possibilities. Kathleen liked helping, like seeing politics used in the old-fashioned way, as an instrument for human need. Because she had a daughter herself, Kathleen knew what Gary was going through. This only increased her determination to find the information or answers he was looking for.

It was May 1st now, and the first words in Teddi's chart that day were "malignant astrocytoma." The words hung there, like a death sentence. Dr. Nelson noted in his report that day that "the tumor looks quite aggressive." He thought she should be referred to the Radiation Therapy team but wrote that "the patient's father would like several opinions about tumor therapy."

Teddi's condition was stable that day. She had several visitors, and gifts started to arrive. Word had gotten around that Teddi, like most children, loved stuffed animals. The number in her collection, consisting mostly of teddy bears, was now close to forty. Despite the newness and glamour of some of the bears, and monkeys, and even a large stuffed St. Bernard dog, Teddietta—bandaged and looking even more worn and torn—remained a constant companion at Teddi's side.

Later that night, after everyone had left, Teddi complained to the nurse that her "stitches and head hurt." The swelling on her face, noted the nurse, seemed to have subsided.

One of the first pieces of information Gary asked Kathleen Rose to investigate was an article, left anonymously on his desk at work, concerning the experiments of a Japanese doctor with a new drug called ACNU. Billed as a "medical breakthrough," the headline read: "Experimental Drug Destroys Brain Tumors." Though the reporter's name was given, there was no clue as to the article's source.

The article told the dramatic story of an eleven-year-old boy who was saved by the drug. "When he came to the hospital he could not stand up by himself," said the researcher, Dr. Yoshikazu Saito of Japan's Tottori University. "He had a brain stem tumor. In two months, with ACNU, there was a huge reduction in the size of the tumor. In 18 months," the report went on, " he became a normal child again, returning to school. Since then he hasn't shown any symptom of the tumor."

Attempting to track down the source of the report, among others, Kathleen contacted the science editor of *The New York Times*. She finally found out that the article was from *The National Enquirer*, and obtained the reporter's phone number. He confirmed the story.

Kathleen told Gary, who was then in Albany himself, about her conversation with the reporter. Gary, in turn, put a call through to Dr. Saito in Japan. What he had forgotten was the time difference and that he couldn't speak a word of Japanese. Dr. Saito answered, groggily, and Gary tried to tell him in English that he was sorry, and that he would try to call back later. Kathleen went to work trying to find someone who could translate for Gary.

On that first day, Kathleen had also called the National Cancer Institute in Bethesda, Maryland. The Institute is charged with developing a coherent and systematic national program in the fight against cancer. It shares information, provides funding for research, and establishes standards for research facilities and treatment centers.

Kathleen forwarded the article appearing in *The National Enquirer* to them. Through the intervention of Barber Conable, a western New York Congressperson and now head of the World Bank, an appointment was arranged for May 17th. It was to be a memorable experience.

Toward the end of the first hectic day, Kathleen also made contact with the chief oncologists at two of the leading cancer centers in the world: the Memorial Sloan-Kettering Cancer Institute in Manhattan; and the Roswell Park Memorial Institute in Buffalo, New York. The last phone call of the day was to the chief of pediatrics at the Hospital of the Albert Einstein School of Medicine. He agreed to review Teddi's records when her stay at Strong Memorial Hospital was over.

Meanwhile, at Strong, a resident had come by to talk to Teddi about her operation. The doctor noted in her report that "Liz" knew she had a tumor and that it could not be completely removed. The doctor added: Teddi also is aware of the X-ray treatments, but is not sure exactly what they are for. She says the "doctors talked about that with my dad." The child, the report also noted, "expressed her desire to know."

Though in the morning she felt unusually tired, clinically she was doing well. There were no complaints of headaches, nor did she vomit. And the surgical wound, according to the nurse's examination of it, seemed to be healing well.

Bob Mervis was sensitive to the fact that at that point Teddi was becoming anxious about missing school. An elementary school teacher, Bob began to tutor his niece, picking up her homework himself after school.

It was May 2nd and Kathleen Rose was trying to locate prominent neurosurgeon Dr. Michael Walker at the Baltimore Cancer Research Center. Walker had moved to the National Cancer Institute, and the assistant to Congressperson Conable was trying to help contact him. Kathleen also telephoned the Child Cancer Study Group at the University of California in Los Angeles for advice regarding Teddi's condition. Experts there suggested she contact Sloan-Kettering and Roswell Park.

Having gotten through to the Chief of Pediatrics at Sloan-Kettering, Kathleen was told that if Gary had all of Teddi's records sent to them from Strong Memorial Hospital, they could then make an appointment. He felt that Dr. William R. Shapiro, a member of the American Association for Cancer Research and the American Society for Clinical Oncology, Inc., would see the Mervises without hesitation.

This part of Gary's campaign had a positive affect on him. He had been cautioned by doctors and others that he may not be able to see these prominent people and yet here they were, ready to review the records of his little girl.

On May 3rd, Kathleen checked on a new radiation and microwave treatment discovered by a doctor in Australia. It was reported to have dissolved tumors or reduced them, and had few side effects, including no hair loss.

Teddi seemed to be making an astonishing breakthrough of her own that day. The nurse reported in her chart that Teddi "looked wonderful" and had no complaints, no headaches, and no dizziness. She was out of bed and walking, and there was no sign of irregularity or weakness. The nurse also noted that because of Teddi's improvement, her Decadron dosage was being tapered. Teddi wanted to know when she could go home.

Later in the day the doctor removed Teddi's sutures. The wound had healed well. He noted in her chart: "Father's wish to seek alternative opinions as to therapy discussed on 'rounds,' and feeling was that this should be supported to an extent in order that he will feel that he has done 'all' for Liz."

The next day, May 4th, Gary drove to Roswell Park in Buffalo. He wanted to deliver Teddi's records himself. He was told that Teddi's pathology and a recommendation for treatment would be prepared as soon as possible.

An appointment for Gary was made at Albany Medical College with Dr. John Horton, head of Oncology. Other professionals Kathleen spoke with suggested she contact Dr. Chu Chang of Columbia/Presbyterian Medical Center. It was located on Manhattan's upper west side. Part of a consortium that included Columbia University, a Cancer Center Institute of Cancer Research was also there. It was one of the three federally designated "Comprehensive Cancer Centers" in New York City. There were only twenty-two in the entire United States.

Both Kathleen and Gary made special note of both physicians and hospitals mentioned more than once. They would take a similar approach later in confirming Teddi's pathology and therapy options.

Kathleen called Dr. Paul Kornblith's office that day to schedule an appointment. Kornblith, with the National Institutes of Health, had been Dr. Nelson's mentor at Massachusetts General Hospital. Nelson was Teddi's neurosurgeon.

Teddi kept progressing. She could sit up in bed, and in a chair. She wanted to and did walk more. Still, there were minor yet worrisome occurrences: one day she had a nosebleed; another day her left pupil was more dilated and slower to react than the right one. Teddi didn't complain about these occurrences, and according to the doctor's report, she seemed neurologically stable.

The doctor told Teddi that she could go home and on May 7th, after nearly two weeks, she left the hospital. With an arm wrapped around Teddietta, and her other hand holding onto her mother's, once outside the hospital Teddi paused momentarily, overwhelmed by the warm air and freedom.

Gary wasn't there to join in the joyous occasion. He had remained in Albany because there had been a break in trying to communicate with Dr. Saito of Japan, the experimenter with the ACNU drug. Kathleen found a Japanese doctor at Albany Medical College who agreed to serve as an interpreter in the proposed conversation with Dr. Saito. She had gone into Professor Hideshige Imai's office without an introduction or appointment.

"Look," she said. "Can you help? We've got a big problem and we think you can help." After explaining the situation, Dr. Imai said he would be glad to help. Kathleen had the overseas operator begin putting the phone call through.

Gary called home and talked with both Sheri and Teddi. He was feeling buoyant. As they waited for the overseas connection to be made, evening fell. Downstairs, in the State Legislative Office Building, a celebration for Republicans was taking place. But Gary, along with Dr. Imai, was on the fifth floor, in Jim Nagle's office, waiting. Irene Matichyn, in town on legislative business, was also present, there to lend moral support. The phone rang. It was Saito.

The questions poured from Gary. Had Dr. Saito published more information about his work with ACNU? He asked about the starting clinical conditions of the tumors Saito studied. Had the doctor divided his study into those who did, and those who did not, have radiation therapy? Could other nitrosourea drugs such as CCNU and BCNU compare with ACNU? What, he wanted to know, were the all-important survival statistics of those treated with ACNU?

Gary was anxious. As soon as Kathleen nodded, indicating she had gotten all of Dr. Saito's remarks, as translated by Dr. Imai, Gary was onto the next question. From there, he gave Dr. Saito a rundown of Teddi's case. He finished with a final question: "Would Dr. Saito treat his daughter?"

Afterward, according to Kathleen's notes of the conversation, Dr. Saito had said his procedure involved surgery and the removal of as much of the malignancy as possible. Then radiation and ACNU as the chemotherapy treatment were applied. Saito said a sample of the drug could be sent to a doctor in this country but that it could not be sold because the FDA had not approved of it yet. The doctor went on to say that ACNU was not on the market even in Japan, and that he used it solely on an experimental basis. As far as the United States was concerned, Saito said the best he could do was recommend that Gary contact Dr. Edward Laws of the Mayo Clinic in Rochester, Minnesota. Saito added that Laws probably would be reluctant to guarantee any cure even if Gary did take Teddi to Japan for treatment.

Imai hung up the phone, and Gary felt his discouragement return. There was a large gap between the headline announcement of a new miracle cure and the qualified comments of Dr. Saito.

The next morning, May 8th, Gary met with Dr. John Horton, Head of Oncology at the Albany Medical College. Horton recommended radiation therapy as the best alternative, though repeating that it could not cure Teddi's condition. He recommended radiation over chemotherapy, but also told Gary that tests were demonstrating that patients treated with radiation and the drug BCNU were doing better after two years than having radiation alone.

For radiation treatment, Dr. Horton recommended radiation oncologist, Dr. Omar Salazar. One of the best in the field, Salazar was at Strong Memorial Hospital. Horton told Gary: "I wish we had the money to bring him here."

Horton had also suggested that Gary contact Dr. Chu Chang at Columbia/ Presbyterian Medical Center. That was the second time Gary heard Dr. Chang's name mentioned, and Kathleen immediately placed a call to him. Chang said he would be willing to look at Teddi's records but that Gary would have to get them released through Strong's medical staff. It was his hospital's policy.

Time was closing in. Teddi's doctors at Strong had told Gary that whatever he decided to do on Teddi's behalf would have to be done quickly, otherwise whatever benefits gained from surgery would be lost. It was also necessary for therapy to begin as soon as possible, before the dreaded tumor started to grow again.

Gary put in a call to Roswell Park. Were they ready with Teddi's diagnosis? Could they suggest a protocol?

The pathologist said Teddi had an astrocytoma, a low- to intermediate-grade tumor, with some rapid growing. He recommended radiation treatment combined with chemotherapy.

"Where should I take Teddi for treatment?" was Gary's next question.

The pathologist recommended Strong Memorial Hospital.

All the frustration came to a head now for Gary. "Give me the chief of neurosurgery," he told the Roswell switchboard operator.

The doctor was on the line. After telling the doctor who he was and what the call was about, he asked the doctor for advice as to what he should do.

"Chemotherapy and radiation," the doctor said.

Gary hung up the phone. "Hold my calls," he said to his secretary. Closing the door, he collapsed in his chair.

In spite of all the phone calls, travel, and worry, he found little consensus or assurance about what was the best course to take. He had looked deeply into the reality behind the headlines, had talked with the best the medical community had to offer, and all he had found was that there was no miracle. In fact, the high priests of medicine were not much better off then he was in being sure about what to do and why.

As parents, he and Sheri would have to make a decision that was going to be extremely painful to Teddi and costly to them; one with no guarantees as to its effectiveness. They were going to have to make what could be the most important decision in their daughter's life, and there was precious little to base it on.

8

The New Terms of Hope

Of the non-experimental therapies available to the Mervises, the first was radiation. Next to surgery itself, radiation was the second most common form of cancer treatment. More than half of all cancer patients received radiation as part or all of their treatment therapy.

The purpose of the treatment is to alter the chemistry of the cancer cells themselves. Radiation causes cells to die immediately, or it can sterilize them, rendering them incapable of reproducing. It is also possible that treated cancer cells would fail to subdivide later, also ending their reproductive process.

A second form of treatment is chemotherapy. This involves the use of drugs. Literally hundreds of drugs have been, and are, being tested for cancer treatment in the United States and around the world. The purpose of chemotherapy is to kill cancer cells quickly. The drug used must also be eliminated from the body quickly for it can damage or destroy healthy cells.

Chemotherapy is not without serious side effects, including nausea, vomiting, hair loss, susceptibility to infection, and "blown veins." These are veins which are hard, chordlike, and useless. Because the drugs are so strong, veins inevitably become damaged or collapse, and blood cannot flow through them. More specific side effects depend upon the particular drug being administered.

The cancer experts Gary talked with at Sloan-Kettering suggested that Gary meet with Dr. Lawrence Ettinger at Strong Memorial Hospital, a specialist in brain tumors in children. Gary set up a meeting. He and Teddi waited for a half hour. Ettinger didn't show, and so, frustrated, they left. A second meeting with Ettinger produced more positive results. Gary was surprised, and pleased, to see Dr. Nelson also attend, on his own.

Even though Ettinger recommended chemotherapy, after the meeting was over both Gary and Dr. Nelson were uncomfortable putting Teddi through the agonizing ordeal of chemical treatment when the proposed benefits were so minimal. "If we do chemotherapy and Teddi goes through a lot of pain and still ends up dying," Gary asked his wife later, "would she have been better off if we hadn't done it at all? Would she have enjoyed the remainder of her life more?"

It was May 9th, and Sheri met with Dr. Omar Salazar, the University of Rochester radiologist recommended by Dr. John Horton, head of Oncology at Albany Medical College. A second appointment was then scheduled for two days later so Gary could meet him as well.

In the meantime, however, Gary had made up his mind. He phoned Salazar even before their meeting, telling him he had decided on radiation therapy. The pathologist at Roswell had recommended it, and so had Drs. Horton, Chang, and Shapiro. The next day, Dr. Edward Laws from the Mayo Clinic would recommend it. Later, specialists at the Brain Tumor Clinic at the University of California would recommend radiation treatment as well.

Salazar sent what's called a "consultation report" to Dr. Nelson. In it, Salazar recommended that Teddi receive 150 "rads" daily, five days a week for seven weeks. This strategy was based upon his observation, noted in the report, that "the tumor is deep, is related to ventricles and is already identified with dural implants." Salazar held out the option of increasing the amount of radiation dosage.

When Salazar met with the Mervises on May 11th, he told them Teddi's tumor was large, that it was an astrocytoma grade III. A grade III, he said, made it an intermediate grade tumor. The doctor believed the tumor to be more than five centimeters in size, with considerable swelling around it. "This is a very unusual tumor," he said. "It normally occurs in people who are quite older. Maybe 50 or 60 years of age."

Salazar looked somewhat like Gary—husky, dark-haired, of medium height. While most of the radiologists Gary had talked with said radiation could not be a cure for Teddi's tumor, Salazar wanted to go for the cure. There would be risks, serious ones, to be sure, but the realization was slowly coming to the Mervises—excluding Teddi—that death was waiting no matter what they tried or failed to try.

Salazar was clear about the risks: hair loss—which was a serious emotional blow to a person at any age but even more so to a person Teddi's age. There was the risk of severe swelling, maybe brain damage. He also told them, almost as an afterthought, that there was no way of telling when or if the tumor would begin growing again.

As they left Salazar's office, the Mervises knew another tough part of their ordeal lay ahead. Now they would have to explain all this to Teddi. They would have to explain radiation therapy again, and why they wanted to go ahead with it, and what might happen to her as the therapy proceeded. And they would somehow have to tell her that despite all their logic and reasonings, despite what she would have to endure, there was no guarantee that radiation treatment would kill the tumor and save her life.

As they drove home that evening each wondered whether Teddi would be able to understand. Would she be overtaken by fear? Would she begin to lose confidence? Lose hope? In the doctors? In her parents? In herself? Would she become so discouraged that she wouldn't care anymore? Wouldn't fight hard to stay alive?

Gary's first campaign had failed to accomplish what he had hoped for, and he knew that now. But he also knew it wasn't for lack of trying. What he sought, to the best of his knowledge, simply did not exist. The door to finding a miracle cure, certitude in treatment, confidence in therapy results, slammed shut.

As the weeks turned into months, Gary would continue to explore developments in the field of cancer research. There would be "interferon," hailed as one of the most promising discoveries of the decade and yet, upon investigation, its promise was more in the future than in the present. There was the attempt to discover the cancer equivalent of a guided missile, designed to harness the body's immune response. There would also be "hypothermia," the heating of tumors, and the controversial laetrile.

Kathleen Rose in Albany would keep trying. She tracked down new leads, and went back over old ones. She would contact "holistic" health centers both in the United States and Canada. She also had a friend, a "psychic healer," whom she asked for help. He touched some things owned by Teddi which her father had dropped by. The healer told Kathleen things about the child he could not have possibly guessed at. But then he became silent, almost withdrawn. Kathleen Rose never revealed what the man told her.

Gary, Kathleen, and others would continue to try. But Gary's heart wasn't in it anymore. Under the circumstances, he felt they had made the best possible decision. Dr. Salazar was good, radiation received widespread support, Strong Memorial Hospital had emerged as a much recommended treatment facility.

Gary thought it best to be at Strong because then he would not have to uproot his family. He thought Teddi would benefit by being around familiar surroundings, by her friends.

As the first phase of the most important campaign in Gary Mervis' life drew to a close, a period of discouragement set in. Others could tell. Skip thought he looked like a "little boy who has lost his way . . . like somebody whose whole world had been turned upside down. He didn't know where things belonged anymore. Where he belonged."

The struggle now, for Gary, his family, and friends, was what to do about hope. They tried to comfort themselves with the hope of a miracle cure. It could come at any time and so it was important to keep Teddi alive as long as possible.

There was great love in Teddi's world. It kept coming, even getting bigger, like a river overflowing its banks. There was also faith in Teddi's world: faith that radiation might provide a cure, faith that researchers would discover something quickly, faith in doctors, the power of love, and God.

In the time ahead, faith would have a more difficult time of it than love. But neither faith nor love would have as hard a time as hope. The things hoped for were extraordinary—and the time was growing exceedingly short.

9

Hard Lesson

"It's like a beam of light," Sheri told her daughter. "It goes into the tumor and it stunts its growth. It burns it, frizzles it up like a leaf that's been left in the sun too long. The tumor stops growing and turns brown. It would still be there but it would be dead."

Teddi nodded, accepting the explanation about what radiation was supposed to do, and what she would have to go through. She began treatment immediately. Every day of the week at 1:30 P.M.. for eight full weeks she went.

Sheri would usually take time off from work to take Teddi. Sometimes Tod, Kim, or Teddi's friends came along as well. Afterward, depending on the time of year, they'd all go to the park, shopping, or to the zoo.

Gary also took Teddi in for treatment. His experience troubled him. Radiation therapy at Strong Memorial Hospital is administered in the Radiation Oncology Department, separate from Pediatrics. This meant that when Teddi went in for treatment, she saw only adults. Never present was a child her age going through what she was going through.

The procedure for radiation therapy was also isolating and intimidating. To prepare the patient for treatment, doctors put a mark on the body where the radiation beam would be literally shot through. The patient is told to lie perfectly still on a table which is then wheeled into a room and left alone. Doctors communicated with the patient via a loudspeaker. The rooms where all this took place looked to Gary like the set on "Star Wars."

Treatment made it difficult for Teddi to attend school. Though her parents arranged for a tutor to come to the house, not being with her friends and doing what they were doing compounded Teddi's growing sense of being left out and alone.

Teddi began to ask questions about God. She wanted to know why God would cause her to have a tumor and go through all that she was going through. She wondered if she was being punished for something she had done or failed to do.

Gary knew religious rationales for situations such as these: that God was testing the person; that God wouldn't give the person more than they could bear. But Gary knew he couldn't tell his nine-year-old daughter who grew up believing in a good and loving God anything close to that.

What he did say was that he thought what happened to Teddi simply happened: it was in the nature of things for people to get sick because something didn't balance right. That's how the tumor got its start; something wasn't working right inside of Teddi. He encouraged her not to ask God why but to ask God for strength and to be there for her when she felt alone.

Gary would later say that afterward, Teddi's dark eyes searched his, wondering if there was more he wanted to say. She'd then say "okay Dad" but it wasn't long, her father remembered, when she asked the very same questions all over again.

Gary focused on the "Serenity Prayer" for Teddi: "God grant me the serenity to accept the things I cannot change, the courage to change the things I can change, and the wisdom to know the difference." He tried to get Teddi to understand the prayer and repeat it. They recited it over and over again before bed. Gary knew she was trying hard to understand, and sometimes when he closed her door he muffled the sounds his crying made.

Fortunately, Teddi didn't have much of a reaction to the radiation treatment. She seemed more tired than usual, but that was about all. Fortunate, too, was the journey the Mervis family made together visiting Dr. Paul Kornblith at the National Institute of Health in Bethesda, Maryland.

Kornblith had reviewed Teddi's records prior to the meeting. While the whole family had come together, only Gary and Sheri met with him that sunny May afternoon. After chatting for a few minutes, Kornblith got down to business. He knew how worried they were and he didn't want to prolong their anxiety and desire to know. "If there was something we could use to save your daughter, that could cure her—I don't care what kind of hell we would have to put her through—we'd do it," he told them. He paused, shrugged his shoulders, adding that there was nothing they could do to save or cure her.

A silence fell over the room. Gary was the first to speak. "How much time does she have left?"

Kornblith answered: "Unfortunately nobody can deal with the quantity issue. I can't tell you whether she's going to live a month, six months, a year, six years. Nobody knows."

The doctor didn't think that was reason to despair, however. "The quality of life she has you can deal with. You can control that. What you should do is take what time you have and try to make it the very best time possible."

The Mervis family stopped at Gettysburg, Pennsylvania, on the return trip home. As he drove, Gary kept thinking about Kornblith's words. As he drove, he thought of the prayer he had encouraged Teddi to memorize and understand. And as he drove, he began to see that the prayer was as much for him as it was for Teddi.

10

The Quality of Time

Upon returning home, one of the first decisions made by Gary and Sheri was to buy Teddi a dog. Gary took out books from the library so Teddi could see all the different kinds there were. Her decision? A bulldog.

"You don't want that thing *really*," her mother wanted to know. Gary told her it was ugly. Still, Teddi insisted it was the dog for her.

Sheri went through the newspaper each night with Teddi until they finally found an ad for a bulldog for sale. Kim went along with Sheri and Teddi to buy the dog. Teddi named it "Sweet'ums," and it was a big, ugly dog which grunted whenever it moved.

Not long afterward, they bought Teddi a horse. Teddi had always loved horses and her parents felt like there was no better time than now to let her have one. They let her play baseball, too, and do just about everything else a nine-year-old would want to do. They worried, too: about whether she'd fall off the horse and hurt her head; whether she'd get hit by a pitch.

The horse and the trip to Disney World which followed later were part of the promise Gary had made to his daughter the night before surgery. He felt it important to keep her spirits up and her will to live strong.

It had been a hard spring. Never before had Sheri and Gary been so deeply hurt or bewildered. Their anxiety level heightened, and sometimes it showed. On the trip to Disney World, for example, at one point Sheri anxiously called Kim over to her. Kim had been roller skating, and now Sheri nervously examined Kim's leg. She thought she saw a bump, something that looked like a tumor.

Kim, like Tod, wondered herself if she and her brother would get cancer too, whether it was something a person inherited, like hair color or body size. As they grew older another set of worries followed: would their children, when they were ready to have children, also become victims of cancer?

Teddi continued to respond well to the radiation treatments. She still wasn't becoming sick afterward, as was thought. The fact that the heavy doses of radiation were not directed at an internal part of her body such as her stomach area or lungs seemed to reduce the likelihood of her vomiting, or having stomach cramps and nausea. She still was tired after treatment and often took an afternoon nap.

The medicine Teddi had to take along with radiation therapy was causing her weight to fluctuate significantly. This troubled Teddi. One time she vomited during a doctor's visit. Salazar found out it wasn't from the radiation, but because she was fasting to lose weight.

Then one of radiation's key side effects occurred. Teddi began to lose her hair. One night, playing cards with her sister and her friend, Teddi tugged on her hair and a handful came out. Surprised, she pulled on her hair in a different place. Startled, Kim and the friend began to laugh.

Teddi turned to her mother for comfort. "I'm going to be bald," she cried.

Sheri reminded her that the doctor predicted this might happen. She also told Teddi the doctor had said it might grow back, too. They would have to wait and see.

"I'm going to be ugly, aren't I?" Teddi said.

Her mother would never accept such a statement from her daughter. "You could never be ugly to me, Teddi," she said, holding her as she cried.

The next day Sheri and her daughter went shopping for wigs. They couldn't find one suitable for Teddi because wigs were made for adults, and none was designed to hide baldness. They did find an over-sized wig that Teddi liked, one that would have to do until they could figure something out. Teddi called it her "Roseanna, Roseanna Danna" wig because it was similar in hair-style to that of the Gilda Radner character on "Saturday Night Live."

Kathleen Rose in Albany mentioned Teddi's problem in finding a child's wig to her ex-husband, a hairdresser. He had a child's wig, which had a pony tail, made up especially for Teddi. Gary took his excited daughter to the Greyhound Bus station where it was shipped.

Sheri also found a pink terrycloth hat for Teddi to wear. It was soft and floppy, and Teddi seemed to like it the best of anything that went on her head. Afterward, after it had become special to Teddi, for the life of her Sheri couldn't remember where she had gotten it and so could never replace it. Teddi kept on wearing it anyway. Sheri said it was washed so many times it lost its shape and became so faded and frayed it began to resemble Teddi's worn-out bear Teddietta.

By the start of summer, Teddi was looking better. Gary had wanted his family to make a commitment to be positive. He told them that as a family they were going to stick together and be there for Teddi. His family was pulling together.

The only practical thing that began to bother Gary during that summer was how hot it was, and the fact that Teddi didn't want to go swimming with the family at nearby Canandaigua Lake or Conesus Lake, as they had done in previous summers. Teddi was ashamed of being bald.

Gary and Sheri talked about getting a pool. Gary thought an above-ground pool would do; Sheri was concerned about the family budget. One early August morning they called a contractor to get an estimate. They liked the bid but the contractor couldn't install it the next morning as Gary had wanted. The telephone and electrical wires were in the way.

"You be back in the morning and I'll have the wires moved," Gary told him.

The contractor came back but didn't bring his crew with him. He was surprised to find the wires moved. Gary had gone to the top at both utilities for help.

Late that month, Teddi was due in the doctor's office. Her radiation treatments were now over, and this examination would be crucial. A CT scan was done and Dr. Salazar noted in Teddi's medical record that the tumor "shows a favorable response at this point and this becomes a critical scan to compare with subsequent treatments." He also noted these troubling signs: slight incoordination upon rapid alternating movements; a little tendency of the right eye to go inwards; evidence of some dry blood in Teddi's right ear canal; and some moderate changes in skin color as a result of the radiation.

Salazar, meeting with the Mervises, told them he was generally pleased with the CT scan results and expressed his hope that she would continue to improve. He told Teddi he expected her hair to grow back. Finally, he said, that if Teddi went back to school and continued to do as well as she was, he wouldn't need to see her until three months from then. He said a repeat CT scan would not be necessary for another six months.

This was the best news Teddi, the Mervises, and their friends had had since before the surgery, which seemed so long ago now. Everyone was excited. When Cheryl DeBiase heard the news, for example, she got into the car and drove from Rochester to Canandaigua Lake, miles away, to tell her husband Skip. She stood on the dock shouting, "Teddi's going to be okay! Teddi's going to be okay!" as Skip, in his boat, sped toward her.

To Gary, Teddi looked good. With the radiation treatment over, her medication was reduced. That meant her weight started to come down. Her spirits revived, she was regaining her confidence, and she was looking more and more like the old Teddi. There was a little more hope in his heart.

Sheri was troubled, however, even though she kept most of it to herself. There was, for one thing, the fact that Teddi seemed to tire so easily. Sheri kept waiting for the dark circles around Teddi's eyes to go away.

Teddi's school friends started to come by. So did some of her parents' friends—Irene Matichyn, Skip and Cheryl, and others. Skip sometimes came with his new yellow Corvette on a Sunday to take Teddi to the grocery store for candy or ice cream, or just cruise the city and countryside. Sometimes he'd buy her things just to get the family in an uproar, like the button Teddi proudly came home with which said: "A Bad Woman Is Good to Find."

One Sunday before Skip left with Teddi, he told Sheri that he and Teddi were going to go out drinking. "We'll be back in three days!" he said, taking Teddi's hand and heading for the door.

"You're not taking my daughter alone with you for three days!" Sheri shouted.

"C'mon, Teddi," Skip laughed, "don't listen to your mother—listen to me!"

They all would laugh more. It seemed to come with the optimism. The radiation treatments were over, the tests were positive, and Teddi was looking like her old self: the bounce was back in her step; the ease was back in her smile; she flirted and was as talkative as she had always been. Those who watched sometimes nodded their heads as if to say: "She beat this thing. . . . Thank God she looks like she beat it." But not once in the presence of Teddi or her parents did these things get said out loud.

Teddi started to drop by and visit the Scobells, the next door neighbors. Teddi had asked for permission to call the Scobells Aunt Betty and Uncle Jim because she felt they were more like family or friends than just neighbors. She would have tea and sometimes play cards. Betty Scobell, silver-haired and in her sixties, also had cancer. "We're going to beat this thing," Teddi said to her once.

Throughout the Autumn, Gary was growing increasingly restless. He was doing the best he could in terms of trying to provide Teddi with quality time. But there still seemed like there was more he could do. He felt the call of yet another campaign, one which would provide Teddi with something that was larger than the moment, maybe even larger than her life, but for the life of him he couldn't figure out what it was.

PART II

New Terms of Hope

11

Back to School

Teddi was anxious to return to school that fall, hair or no hair. She liked to learn, read avidly on her own, and often completed assignments long before they were due. Teddi also liked to socialize, and school was a great social experience for her.

Sheri talked with Teddi's teacher. She had learned that he had recently lost two brothers to cancer and was worried about how he would react to Teddi. She feared he would either consciously or unconsciously keep Teddi at arm's length, afraid of getting close to still another person who would die.

Sheri began by telling Edward Dwyer that if Teddi had a seizure one of her girlfriends would take her to the nurse's office. Teddi would have phenobarbitol with her and it would, she told the teacher, in all likelihood make the seizure stop.

Dwyer, in his late forties, listened patiently. He nodded his head from time to time in understanding.

"I'm concerned," Sheri said finally, "that the recent deaths in your own family might somehow reflect on Teddi. That it might be hard for her *and* for you."

This time Dwyer shook his head. No, he told her, the death of his brothers hadn't frightened him or turned him cold; it made his capacity to love grow even more.

Edward Dwyer would be a good teacher and friend to Teddi. Teddi would talk about him to her girlfriends, saying that when she grew up, she wanted to be a teacher just like Mr. Dwyer.

The role of educators and the educational system as both related to childhood cancer would concern the Mervises from that time forward. Sheri's feeling was that anything being structured into the educational system would only serve to draw attention to the child.

Gary, however, felt that educators, and the child's peers, ought to be educated about what children with cancer deal with and endure. He thought there ought to be some preparation of teachers themselves in regards to cancer, its consequences, and what could physically and emotionally be expected in regards to a child with cancer. Gary thought perhaps specific science units could be devoted to cancer and its treatment. He also believed that if children with cancer were encouraged to talk about their illness, their fears might dissipate, and the fears of their peers might dry up and whither away as well. Gary believed that when shielded from reality fears became exaggerated, especially among children, and especially among those with cancer and the people they came into contact with.

Dr. Harvey Cohen, chief of the department of Pediatrics/Oncology at Strong Memorial Hospital, opted for a place somewhere in the middle of where Sheri and Gary stood. Cohen believed in "qualified truth." This meant that children were told difficult information only when they were ready to hear it, only when they gave clues that they wanted to listen. He also believed such information had to be couched in phrases and with feelings children could understand in regard to their own particular stage of development.

As the day marking the beginning of school approached, summer optimism regarding Teddi's condition began to wane somewhat. The dark circles under Teddi's eyes remained. The radiation had affected her skin even more severely than the earlier blotches. Now, especially on her neck, the skin peeled and looked pitted. Lowering her Decadron dosage had made Teddi extremely thin. One day Sheri noticed that Teddi's handwriting had also changed.

Teddi's writing sloped, first from the left, then to the right, then back again. The various letters of a single word might be leaning in several directions at the same time. It bothered Sheri, and it bothered her daughter, too.

"I can't control it," Teddi told her mother, exasperated.

Sheri told her not to worry about it, that it was legible enough to be read.

The night before that first day of school, Sheri told Teddi she would take her the next morning. Teddi disagreed, something she didn't do all that often. She wanted to go on the school bus with her friends. After some debate, Sheri relented.

The following morning, Teddi waited for the bus at the usual stop with her girlfriends and other kids who were waiting as well. She was adjusting the pink hat Sheri had bought to hide her bald head when suddenly one of the boys began to pull on it. But Teddi's friends stuck up for her and the boy stopped.

Teddi's brother, Tod, also attended the same school. Though not a big kid, he was an awfully tough one. After hearing about what happened to Teddi, he went around the hallways telling others that if they picked on his sister they would have him to deal with.

And if that wasn't enough, Teddi's sister Kim heard her mother talking about the incident that night. She told Teddi to let her know if anything like that happened again. She told some potential troublemakers the following morning: "Be cool or I'll have to do something about it"—though she was not quite sure what.

Kim Mervis would seem to have a more difficult time dealing with her sister's illness than her brother Tod. Only a year older than Teddi, she was also popular and very pretty. These things compounded normal sibling rivalries; cancer would compound them even more.

Kim had been a thoughtful caretaker of Teddi at the hospital. But it had seemed easier to her there, with Teddi clearly in pain, with her head bandaged and tubes tied to her. At home, with Teddi somewhat back to normal, the edge seemed off and the rivalry heightened. In one of her angry moments Kim had told Teddi, as if she didn't know already, "You have cancer!"

Fortunately for Kim, she met another girl her age at school that year who had a sister with cancer. She was going through many of the same things Kim was going through and they would talk, tell each other secret fears and worries, become friends. Finding friends was another nice thing both girls were able to do through school.

12

New Hope

The time for Teddi to go to school came and went, and she seemed to do well through the adjustment process. Gary, however, still struggled with the feeling that there was more he could and should be doing. Churning over in his mind was Dr. Kornblith's advice that the giving of quality time itself would be the most important thing. Also churning inside Gary's mind was the same request he'd heard time and again from friends and strangers alike who wanted to do something more for him and for children like Teddi. What was it, they wanted to know. What could they do?

That fall Gary made his first contact with one of Rochester's long-established cancer organizations. Gary had talked to a friend of his about sharing the massive amount of material he had accumulated regarding the pathology and treatment of brain tumors in children. He thought the information might be helpful to other mothers and fathers who were being told their child had a brain tumor.

The organization, when Gary approached it, asked him to serve on its public relations committee. He accepted the assignment even though his real interest was to more directly help the children and the parents of the children with cancer. Though at times discouraged, Gary continued to look for a way to fulfill this desire.

Then, early one December morning as Gary was getting ready to make a political trip to Albany, New York, he heard words coming from the small TV set in the corner of the room that made him slowly come to a stop. Tom Brokaw, NBC's "Today Show" host, was speaking: " . . . And when we come back from this commercial break, we're going to be talking to some very special children."

Gary walked to the edge of the bed, sat, and waited for the program to continue. He left his tie unfastened. The word "special" had drawn him like a magnet, for the word is often used to describe children who are severely handicapped or terminally ill.

The story was about a Camp Special Days in Jackson, Michigan, for boys and girls with cancer. Children with cancer played near the reporter as he told how they often couldn't go to a "regular" camp with "regular" kids because most camps aren't equipped to deal with their special needs. The result, said the reporter, was that children with cancer were excluded from most summer camps.

Camp Special Times, however, was different. Its only purpose was to serve children with cancer. The children themselves got on the air to talk about how much fun they were having swimming, hiking, camping, and meeting other kids like themselves. They didn't appear to be self-conscious, Gary thought, as he watched, and they didn't seem to be at all worried if they were to get sick or even if they couldn't do things some of these other "special" children could do.

This was what he had been waiting for; he knew it instinctively, the match between his skills and his desire to do more. It would be something practical and positive. He could think of little more on his drive to Albany.

Once arriving, he called the "Today Show" and they put him in contact with the Camp Special Times reporter, Eric Burns. Through Burns, Gary contacted some of the key people at the Michigan camp, and finally Dr. George L. Royer, Camp founder.

They spoke that morning and several times over the next weeks and months ahead. By Christmas, Gary had accumulated an extensive amount of information about the Camp, and he added this to his earlier notes and documentation regarding Teddi's tumor.

Teddi's medical condition remained stable. Dr. Salazar would note in his report, following Teddi's examination, that she was "doing remarkably well." He noted that some of her hair was growing back. He shared this with the Mervises, including Teddi, and said they would have to do another CT scan in February. If there were no changes in Teddi's condition by then, they wouldn't have to meet for another month.

Mervis friends and family were present at dinner on Christmas Day. Afterward, Gary told them about his plan to start a summer camp for children with cancer in New York State. People listened, asked questions, and some shook their heads saying there was too much to do and so little time to do it.

Sheri Mervis may have been the only person listening that day who had no doubts that Gary would have a camp in place for children with cancer the following summer. She knew her husband well, knew his passions as well as his relentless ambition to succeed.

Gary contacted his friend Skip DeBiase to tell him what he had in mind. Skip listened carefully, thinking to himself that this was just like Gary, trying to take a negative situation and make something positive, something good, come out of it.

When Gary finished, Skip told him he thought it was a good idea. "Two, maybe three years down the road," he said, "yeah—I can see it happening."

Gary shook his head. "You don't understand. I want to have the camp for this summer."

Skip didn't think it was possible but didn't have a chance to say so. "Can I count on you?" Gary was asking, and Skip couldn't find it in himself to say no.

Later, as Gary began to spend more and more of his time trying to get the Camp started, and as Skip himself became increasingly involved, he would worry about his business, about the time taken from it. But Skip is also a philosophical person. So when the doubts rose within him, he made himself think about all the good the Camp would do and this rekindled his faith that everything else would balance out in the end.

The day after Christmas, Gary made a presentation to the cancer organization's executive committee. He solicited the organization's help in establishing a camp for children with cancer in the Rochester area. They asked him to make the same presentation to their board of directors.

Dr. Royer was on the phone with Gary and invited him to see the camp in Michigan. Gary thought that perhaps it would be best if Royer came to Rochester, bringing his slides and literature with him, as part of an effort to start a similar camp. Royer said he would be pleased to come, and the cancer organization in Rochester made arrangements, setting the date for Thursday, January 17th, at eleven A.M.

Gary did the legwork of getting people to attend the meeting. He sent out invitations; he followed them up with a phone call. Sande Macaluso was in Gary's office the morning the telephoning began. A deputy marshall and one of Monroe County's Civil Defense officers, Macaluso helped make the phone calls along with others who had dropped by.

Gary would begin nearly every conversation with the words: "Hey, do you remember when you asked me if there was anything you could do?" He said it over and over again, to each person he called, and after they answered "yes" he'd tell them now what they could do.

He talked of the proposed camp for children with cancer that he wanted to see realized by summer; he asked them to make a commitment to hear Dr. Royer talk and to see what had been done for children with cancer in Michigan.

January 17th arrived, and more than 100 people had come to hear Royer's talk. Royer himself was surprised at the turn-out, and the positive publicity which preceded his visit. Not all of those who had come were friends or acquaintances of Gary and his wife. Some had read about this young dream in the newspaper and had come to see if they too wanted to be a part of seeing it realized.

One such person was Polly Schwensen, a pediatric social worker at Strong Memorial Hospital. In her late twenties, Polly worked with children with cancer and their families.

Polly's father died while she was young; her mother had had polio. Her choice of profession, and what to do within it, was based upon a strong philosophical conviction that no one knew how long they were going to live, and that all life, however brief, should be afforded the same opportunity for love and happiness. Polly Schwensen also possessed a deep and abiding faith in God.

After Royer's presentation, Polly made her way to the front of the room. She was angry with something she had heard and wanted to challenge it. Challenging did not come easy to her, and so as she struggled to get Royer's attention, she could feel her heart pounding and her face becoming flushed.

"Excuse me, sir," she said, and Royer turned in her direction. Her tone silenced those around him.

"You said in your talk that you didn't want any social workers at your camp because all they wanted to do was analyze the kids, and that made the kids uncomfortable and homesick for their parents." She paused, knowing that she was talking too rapidly and too loudly. "You said you'd rather see the kids go off and have fun."

Everybody was looking at her now. The only thing that kept her from fleeing at that point was the respect she had for her profession and her life in it.

Royer seemed surprised. "I'm not saying all social workers are like that," he said. "But this has been my experience."

What Polly said next was right from the heart: "I just wanted you to know that there are a few of us who see ourselves differently. If you write off the whole social work population, then you're writing off people who can help you out."

At the next cancer organization meeting, a commitment was made to set aside $12,000 from the budget to establish a summer camp for children with cancer. Gary knew he would have to somehow raise three times that amount in the short time ahead to make the proposition viable.

Still, this was a beginning, and in the midst of winter Gary felt a new burst of energy within him. He was not on the sidelines now, he was in the arena. He was about to launch a second campaign.

To organize the camp, Gary turned to some key people, among them attorney Tom Gosdeck. Gary had helped Tom find a job when he was first out of law school; now Tom proved invaluable in handling all legal matters associated with the camp. Doug Brown, a college buddy of Gary's, took charge of the day-to-day operations of the camp. Fran Russo, chief fiscal officer for Monroe County Human Services, and Raymond Cordello, Controller of the County, developed a budget, and established bookkeeping procedures. Dr. Klemperer was key, as was Sande Macaluso—ready to take care of the camp's many details without hesitation or complaint. Ms. Adele House handled correspondence, typed letters, and made telephone calls. Jack Slattery, a man with an impressive newspaper background, took care of press releases. Volunteering his time, in the process Slattery would find new meaning in a long life.

Young attorney Tom Gosdeck looked around at what was happening and saw something providential in it all. Gary's range of friends had always been wide, from the city's political leaders, to those who fixed the roads. "It was like it was already planned," Tom thought to himself, "all planned somewhere years ago. It had to be Gary Mervis."

Some key organizations made an initial commitment, and that made it somewhat easier to lean on others. The Northeast Kiwanis Club in Rochester held a huge benefit, which included all the Kiwanis organizations in the Greater Rochester Area, on behalf of the proposed camp. The Pittsford Welcome Wagon was an initial, and sustained supporter.

The first priority of the founding organizers of the camp was to decide on a name. Gary thought that the children attending would come when they were reasonably well or feeling good. He also hoped their experience with camp would be a special one. Combining the two sentiments he came up with "Camp Good Days and Special Times." Though there was initial resistance to the name, mainly because of its length, the name stuck.

Then Gary received a phone call from Joseph "Bello" Snyder. In his late sixties, Snyder received the nickname as a Jewish kid growing up in an Italian neighborhood. "Bello" means "beautiful" in Italian, and Snyder used the word often when he spoke; sometimes he made the "Sign of the Cross" when he was particularly moved by something.

"Gary," said the elderly man, "I remember you from high school. Remember me?"

Gary remembered. Bello had been a local basketball star and then played professionally for a decade before retiring. Since that time he had owned and operated a private summer camp for boys and girls. Gary knew it was somewhere in the Adirondacks.

"Look, Gary," said Bello, "I read about you and your daughter in the newspaper, and how you want to have this camp for children with cancer. It touched my heart." Bello paused. "Beautiful," he said, then repeated the word. "I'd like to meet with you and tell you a little about the camp I own."

Bello was in Rochester and so the two met the following day. Gary learned that Snyder's place was called Camp Eagle Cove and was on the south shore of Fourth Lake in Inlet, New York. He showed Gary color photographs of the Camp, with its cabins, indoor bathrooms, big recreation hall, athletic fields for archery, horseback riding, tennis, basketball, and baseball. The Camp also had an excellent waterfront, Bello said, and boating would be a fun thing for the kids. He also pointed out that things of interest for children such as the "Enchanted Forest" amusement park, the Adirondack Museum, and Lake Placid, were all close enough for day trips.

As Gary listened and looked over the photographs, he knew Bello's camp would be perfect for them. In addition to all the features Bello had named, it was beautiful, pollen-free, and one of the more choice camping spots of those in New York and many other states.

Snyder was pleased with Gary's response. He leaned across the table now, wanting there to be no mistake in what he was about to say. He then told Gary he wanted to donate the entire fifty-five-acre facility to the children for one week the following summer. Gary was too surprised to respond but Bello could tell by Gary's expression that he would accept his offer. "Beautiful," said Bello. "Beautiful."

Not long after that, Dr. Robert Cooper, head of the University of Rochester Cancer Center searched Gary out. "You're going to have your camp, Mr. Mervis," he said. "We're behind it here at the hospital."

Dr. Martin R. Klemperer, chief of Pediatric Hematology/Oncology at the University of Rochester, then approached Gary. The Mervises had never met him because Teddi received her radiation treatments in a part of the hospital separate from pediatrics.

Klemperer, medium-sized with thinning hair, ardently wanted to see people's attitudes toward children with cancer changed. The prevailing view, he thought, was medieval and prevented such children from experiencing much of what could be normal in their lives. He felt prejudice warped the thinking of others, including that of parents of children with cancer, further diminishing a child's chance of enjoying a piece of their childhood.

Dr. Klemperer wanted to help others understand that just because a child had cancer, that did not necessarily mean they were bed-ridden or had to be treated in an over-protective manner. Children with cancer were physically capable of doing many of the same things children without cancer were capable of doing.

The doctor introduced himself to Gary. He told him of his roles at the hospital, and that he had heard about Gary's desire to have a camp for children with cancer. He then asked Gary if the camp had a medical director.

"No," Gary answered.

"You do now, Mr. Mervis," Klemperer said.

13

The Second Campaign

It was February and Teddi had to go in for still another CT scan. The doctors advised that this was an important one, for enough time had elapsed after surgery, and radiation treatment, to tell if the tumor was again growing. While there was every reason to be confident, those nagging doubts continued to haunt the Mervises. They thought about the fact that Teddi had not *completely* returned to normal, either in appearance or coordination. The fact that the tumor was still inside Teddi's brain was always cause for worry.

Dr. Nelson's voice, normally reserved, sounded excited when he called the Mervis home with the results. "It shows remarkable improvement over the CT scan of six months ago," said Nelson, much to the surprise and delight of Gary and his wife.

A month later, Teddi went for a medical examination with Dr. Salazar. He wrote in her chart for that day:

> I have performed a total neurological examination on this patient and the only abnormal finding that I was able to detect was incoordination with the left hand and clumsiness particularly when doing rapid alternating movements. Upon questioning the parents, she has been favoring the right hand ever since her original operation.

But there was even more good news. Unless there was a dramatic change in Teddi's condition, Salazar told all three, there was no need to see her until May. Though outside his office the March winds howled and fought the onset of the sun, it didn't seem to matter to Teddi and her parents. They knew spring was coming, they could feel it in their bones, and with it the warm air of hope.

These hopeful developments in Teddi's condition gave fire to her father.

In order to raise money for the camp, he was often out late four or five nights a week that spring and early summer. He spoke whenever he was asked, and went wherever he was invited. He spoke with people at breakfast meetings, at lunch, and after dinner; he talked with people over the phone and across the table.

His campaign was turning into a crusade. He knew it; and others could feel it. He wasn't only out there on the campaign hustings to raise money to establish a summer camp for children with cancer, he was proclaiming to the world that the isolation, the prejudice, the downright humiliation of children with cancer was at an end.

Gary Mervis' message was in essence always the same; the "stump" speech of the active campaigner.

"In our society," he'd begin, "we tend to treat children with cancer differently. Teachers, neighbors, friends—and especially families—look upon them differently. There is always that over-protective hand on the shoulder. And," he'd say, nodding for emphasis, "I've been just as guilty of this as the next father—or mother.

" . . . But I'm convinced that what all these children with cancer want is just the same as what other children their own age want: they want to have fun, they want to live a little dangerously, they want to be with their peers. For most kids with cancer there is a time of remission, when there are no bandages or any other reason why they can't go out and play with their brothers and sisters, roller-skate and ride a bike. Inside they want to know why they can't be out there too; why they can't be playing the same way too."

Gary would normally reach deep inside himself then, to that beautiful spring day not more than a year ago when his entire world collapsed under him, the false promises of a miracle cure, the long nights of worry and waiting.

"Attitude is important," he'd tell people, "if you have a positive attitude, then you will begin to realize that it isn't the length of somebody's life that matters—it's the quality of that life. . . . And I'll tell you something: when I began to think this way then the entire idea of starting a summer camp for children with cancer began to make a lot of sense."

Gary loved it, every discouraging and uplifting minute of it. He had run other people's campaigns, listened to hundreds of others speak, and now it was his turn, his campaign, his speech. There were moments when out of exasperation he wondered if it was all worth it: somebody would plan to have him speak, he would make the trip, only to arrive and find somebody forgot to send out an announcement. There were moments when he was so tired he didn't think he would be able to get out of bed the next morning to begin again.

But this campaign wasn't for his own election or re-election, it wasn't for his own gain, it was for Teddi and those like her. He was a champion for the children, suffering children. To Gary, and to others, it was the highest of causes—maybe the only cause, which truly mattered. This is a world in which children suffer, Albert Camus had said, and all we can do is lessen the number of suffering children. And if we do not do this, then who in the world will do this?

Teddi sometimes joined her father on the campaign hustings. Though he didn't feel he could bring any child with cancer along, and had misgivings about bringing a child at all, he also believed that people who would give their time, money, or both, expected something in return, even if it was a handshake or a smile. Additionally, Gary wanted to educate audiences about childhood cancer, to let them see that children with cancer were loving, vital human beings and that there was nothing horrifying or grotesque about them as many people believed. He wanted audiences to see that children with cancer did not have to be, nor deserved to be, shut away from the activity of the world—locked away as if they were mentally ill or physically dangerous.

Sheri would enjoy watching the two of them leave together, hand-in-hand, out the door. "She acts just like a little old lady," thought Sheri, "telling her father what to wear and what to watch out for."

After several such joint appearances, they were riding home together one night, and Gary told Teddi what a good impression she was making on people, how much she was doing for children with cancer.

"Gee, Dad," said Teddi, "I really am important, aren't I?"

There was no mistaking for Teddi that the idea for the camp, and what her father and others were doing, was not for her alone. A reporter asked Teddi: "What do you think about all your father is doing for you?"

Teddi told him straightaway: "Oh, he's doing it for all the kids with cancer."

By mid-summer the hundreds of details associated with opening up and running the camp were being hammered out. The medical staff, headed by Dr. Klemperer and other specialists from the University of Rochester Medical Center, Buffalo's Roswell Park Memorial Institute, and Upstate Medical Center in Syracuse, New York, considered first the feasibility of medical supervision, and then plans to implement it.

Counselors were recruited and training sessions held. Each was given a manual containing their responsibilities and duties, and they would read and reread it to make sure they had it right, for it was all new to them. One passage they talked about was written by H. Q. Cooper. Originally intended to describe what it took to be a successful teacher, members of the staff thought it applied to counselors as well. Individuals would need, said the passage:

> The education of a college president.
> The executive ability of a financier.
> The craftiness of a politician.
> The humility of a deacon.

The discipline of a demon.
The adaptability of a chameleon.
The hope of an optimist.
The courage of a hero.
The wisdom of a serpent.
The gentleness of a dove.
The patience of a Job.
The grace of God—And
the persistence of the devil.

A Rochester area newspaper, publicizing the need for counselors, described the work in a unique "Help Wanted" format:

Responsibilities—frightening. Work—very hard.
Hours—interminable. Working conditions—beautifully wooded campsite on a lake in the mountains. Job opportunities—a multitude. Financial remuneration—non-existent. Compensation—boundless. Most important qualification—unlimited capacity to love.

In addition to the medical staff and counselors, a waterfront director had to be found; specialists in arts, crafts, archery, games, woodworking, riflery, and other sports also had to be recruited. They also needed a kitchen staff and drivers to take the children from the three launch sites in Buffalo, Syracuse and Rochester to the campsite. Athletic and camping equipment had to be purchased, meals planned, and dozens of special programs and events mapped out and organized. Details ranged from whether there would be enough money to run the burgeoning operation to how many pounds of spaghetti would be needed for Wednesday's dinner.

A little more than a week before Camp was to start, Teddi had another CT scan, as well as another medical examination by Dr. Salazar. The scan showed no evidence of recurrent disease, though Teddi complained of an occasional headache, particularly when she jumped up and down, seizures sometimes occurred and there was the troublesome motor incoordination. Dr. Salazar noted in his report that "the neurologic and physical examinations are in status quo." Also in his report was mention of the fact that some members of a TV crew had come with Teddi, and her mother and father that day, as part of a story about Teddi to publicize the Camp. Dr. Salazar wished Teddi luck at Camp.

As Gary's interest and commitment to the development of a Camp grew, he found himself drawing more and more away from the goals of the local cancer organization of which he had been a part.

Their emphasis was on raising money to fund research, buy equipment, and to look for a cure. While Gary agreed this had to be done, and a cure for cancer had to be found, he also believed that something needed to be done in regard to improving the life of those who had the disease.

The deadline for the Camp's opening was near and Teddi began to have mixed emotions about it. Gary and the screening committee were reviewing applications for the Camp, and along with their medical histories, the children were asked to submit photographs of themselves. The Camp staff thought this would be a good way to come to know the children even before they arrived. Sometimes, Gary brought a few of these pictures home with him to show to Teddi, to ease her anxiety.

The more Teddi saw, the more excited she would become: they would be kids like her, with cancer, not always feeling well, some without hair and sometimes even without an arm or leg. They would be going through the same thing she was; they would know what her world was like from the inside. She didn't know and had never seen so many others with which she had so much in common.

But her excitement alternated with her nervousness. "Do you want to go to camp, Mommy?" she'd sometimes asked, out of nowhere. "I don't want to go without you," she'd follow up saying.

Sheri tried to comfort and reassure Teddi, telling her that she would definitely come, and so would a lot of other people she knew, and kids just like her who would be nervous, too. They would love her, too, just like she did, regardless of whether she had hair, tired easily or was afraid.

As the Camp's opening date, August 29th, closed in, Camp organizers and chief sparkplug, Gary Mervis, moved at a feverish pace. When they talked, the atmosphere became emotionally charged—electric.

Gary was raising funds and educating right to the very end. These final days of the campaign found Gary's voice hoarse, his body exhausted. It was all a matter of heart now.

"Vanity has no age," he would tell audiences. "The bodies of children with cancer go through a lot of changes: these children get tired, they vomit, they lose their hair, they have excessive bleeding. These children become self-conscious about these things, and often withdraw. But at Camp Good Days," he'd say, smiling, for he knew it was going to happen now, "at Camp Good Days and Special Times such hardships will be the rule, not the exception!

". . . Other children with cancer are probably the only ones who really know what it's like. When my daughter had to go through eight weeks of painful radiation treatment last summer, never once did she meet up with another child. She never had a confidante of her own age who was going through what she was going through, who had the same fears, and worries, and words.

"We say we understand, we adults, but we really don't. Not in the same way and with the same words as somebody their own age. The isolation children with cancer have to needlessly endure and what happens to them mentally and emotionally is as debilitating as what happens to them physically."

The City's afternoon newspaper, the *Rochester Times-Union*, carried an editorial about the Camp's opening. Entitled "A Dream Come True," the editorial stated that childhood cancer patients have been a "forgotten group, but no longer, thanks to [Gary] Mervis . . . "

There was only one thing that began to gnaw at the organizers, Gary chiefly among them. It started slowly, was somewhat vague, and then grew to an obsession. In reality, would the parents of children with cancer actually let them go? Would they let these children travel some two hundred miles for one week with strangers taking their place?

These were big questions, crucial questions now, and there was nothing to do but hope, pray, and try to reassure one another that something so good and important couldn't help but succeed.

14

Waiting and Letting Go

Gary drove to the campsite on Wednesday, August 27, two days before camp was to open. Other members of the staff, including safety head Sande Macaluso, were also there. Counselors, too, began arriving.

Gary phoned Sheri that night. Like Sheri, he personally was not much of a camping enthusiast. He had not done it while growing up, and he wasn't at all certain he was going to like it now. So far, he told his wife, he didn't like it much.

"God, Sheri," he told her, "there are all these noises at night. I'm not sure if there are bears outside the cabin—but I am sure there are mice inside!"

Sheri laughed.

"I'm going to get my .38!" Gary joked.

"And do what," Sheri joined in, "shoot 'em?"

The counselors who had arrived went into town that night. On the way in, conversation turned to Adirondack bears. Some claimed to have seen them, big ones, that could run with the speed of a track star. Others thought these were just tall tales—stories people told around the campfire at night.

About 3:00 A.M. that morning, the female counselors, sleeping in one cabin, were startled by noises coming from outside. They heard growling and were about to scream for security when they heard laughter as well. It seems as though the male counselors wanted to do some convincing about the Adirondack bears.

Sheri drove to the campsite the following morning. Tod, Kim, and Teddi were with her. Teddi's anxiety mounted: What would they think of her hat? Would other kids be bald? She also asked if she could stay with her mother, in her cabin, rather than with other children.

Though Sheri didn't let on, she was also nervous—about Teddi being there at all, about what might happen in the week ahead after all the planning, the fund-raising, the work. This was a first time for her, and she and her staff would be responsible for everything from blowing up 5,000 balloons to feeding more than 100 children, counselors, staff, and all the guests who were sure to come by.

Sheri, like her husband, was also a little nervous about the camping experience itself. She would, that night, nonchalantly shake out her sleeping bag. She wanted to make certain there were no mice inside of it!

More of the counselors arrived the morning Sheri had come including Ann Kiefer, who was to be Teddi's counselor that week. Kiefer, articulate and tenacious, kept a journal about her feelings and the experience of that week. One of her entries dealt with seeing Teddi.

> ... I had my first glimpse of Teddi. She was smaller than I thought she'd be, but so pretty, with her button nose, long, dark lashes and sweet mouth. She wore a long-billed pink hat to hide her baldness, and that hat, with its ridiculous brim, was like her trademark all week. She disappeared after the meeting with her parents but returned to the cabin later to sleep.

That afternoon Doug Brown and Assistant Program Director Jan Bruczicki called all the counselors together and went over their duties and responsibilities. Brown, assistant director of student activities at Monroe Community College, emphasized the self-discipline they would need. At no time, he said, was a youngster to be on his or her own without supervision. That didn't mean hovering over them, but it did mean keeping them within eyesight. Most of the kids, he said, had no camping experience whatever.

Brown paused. When he spoke again his voice was intense. "Now pay attention to this," he told the counselors. "One thing I want to happen tomorrow when the children come is for you to drop everything you're doing and be out there to greet them! I want you to come running! Not just running—but whooping and hollering! The noisier the better. Those kids are going to know right from the start that they are welcome here and we're here for them. . . . And that's an order!"

Dr. Klemperer then rose to speak. "Welcome to you all," he began, in the soft, low-key way he had. "I just wanted to tell you where the infirmary is—and I also want to tell you not to rush in there every time one of our kids stubs their toe. Nobody would be doing that at a so-called 'normal' camp—and we won't be doing it here."

Other last minute information and changes were given to counselors and staff. After that, they were free to roam the campgrounds, though most made last minute preparations for the arrival of tomorrow's campers. The staff, too, worked to complete last-minute details of the Camp's opening.

Margaret Register, who was known as "Muggs"—a name she picked up as a kid growing up—would work at the waterfront that year, as well as be a cabin counselor. She looked as young as some of the campers and had their youthful enthusiasm as well. Though she wouldn't get to know either Teddi, or the Mervises very well that summer, she would play an important role in Teddi's life later on.

Social Worker Polly Schwensen had also volunteered to be a counselor. She was determined to show Royer, and those who thought like him, that social workers could do more than analyze and make recommendations about individual behavior; she believed she could demonstrate that they were caring, empathetic professionals. She had a setback of sorts when she introduced herself to Gary, who said he didn't think much of social workers because of his past experiences with them. It stiffened her resolve to make a difference at Camp Good Days and Special Times.

Skip and Cheryl DeBiase also came. They had become even closer to the Mervises because of Teddi's ordeal and now gave up a week's vacation to pitch in and help. Cheryl joined Sheri's staff in the kitchen, but Skip, at least in the beginning, had no assigned role and remained uncertain as to how he might best be of help.

That night, Sande Macaluso again drove from the campgrounds to the Faxton Hospital in Utica. Sande was responsible for Camp security and safety, and he was a conscientious, worried staff member. If a fire were to break out at Camp, or any other such calamity occurred, Sande would take it personally and hard. After all, strangers had entrusted him and the others with their children, children who were seriously ill. Sande had checked with the Inlet police and fire departments arranging for communications, even setting up a "hot line" to each. He traveled and timed the routes they would have to take to the Camp in case of an emergency.

The next morning, far from camp, parents got their children ready and drove them to the bus departure points in Buffalo, Rochester and Syracuse. Eyewitnesses said that parents and children both experienced emotions ranging from terror to exhilaration. One particular boy experienced both.

The boy was reluctant to go at all. Once his parents arrived at the Rochester departure point, he was afraid to leave them and board the bus. After his parents convinced him he would be all right, he arrived at Camp and immediately wrote them a postcard saying he was having a terrible time and to please come and get him. A half hour later he got Sande Macaluso to fish his postcard out of the mailbox because he was having the best time of his life.

Three girls, unknown to each other, were also coming that morning and were to play a significant role in Teddi's life. One was Suzie Parker, from Camden, New York, which was near the city of Rome, who was being driven to the Syracuse departure point. When she was five years old, Suzie was diagnosed as having leukemia. But that didn't prevent Suzie from taking ballet lessons, being active in school acrobatics, or enjoying horseback riding.

Laurie Allinger was being driven that morning to the Rochester departure area, as was Laurie Kaleta, known to her friends as "Froggy" because she loved the water so much. Laurie Allinger, diagnosed a few years earlier as having bone cancer, had to have her right arm amputated at the shoulder almost immediately. Whereas Suzie Parker's appearance seemed normal, there was no hiding Laurie's loss of an arm.

The amputation caused Laurie Allinger several months of pain and depression. Sometimes kids at school made fun of her. Whenever she went out people stared, or their eyes darted away whenever Laurie caught them staring. Laurie Allinger and Laurie Kaleta would later talk about the fact that they never saw other children with cancer, even though—like Teddi—they had gone to Strong Memorial Hospital frequently for treatment. They wished they could have have met there.

Laurie Kaleta, or "Froggy," especially wanted to meet Teddi. She had seen Teddi's name, and sometimes her picture, on Camp brochures. She had even seen Teddi on television once or twice. She said she wanted to meet Teddi because Teddi had "such a kind face."

Then the buses filled with children of varying thoughts, emotions, and expectations left Buffalo, Rochester, and Syracuse and began to head to the campsite. The Buffalo bus would have to travel some 200 miles; the other two buses were progressively closer. Aboard each bus was a Camp staff member. On the bus leaving from Rochester was the young attorney, Tom Gosdeck.

Tom said the kids on the bus were quiet at first. Then they got to know each other a little but still it was quiet—at least for a busload of children. But then out of nowhere a kid yelled, "We're going to Camp!" and there was pandemonium. All their fears, anxieties, and uncertainties seemed to come uncorked, and they kept up their racket all the way to the Camp. Laurie Allinger remembered calling out the window, calling out over and over again, "Are we there yet?! How much longer?!"

Suzie Parker's ride from Syracuse followed the same pattern, and was just as spirited, despite the fact that their bus broke down. Another bus was called and they seemed to handle the misfortune with the resilience which perhaps only these children could truly know.

It was quite an adventure, even the bus ride. They were going to a place they had never been before, at least not together, and with other kids like themselves. And they were going to a camp that was the first of its kind in the northeastern United States. Those days, months, and sometimes years of being stared at, being different, being left out of things melted away along with the miles.

That morning, before the children were due to arrive, the Camp staff, counselors, and all others who had come began to gravitate to the playing fields. This was where the buses would pull in. "We listened," Anne Kiefer wrote in her journal, "...we listened for every car or truck that passed, thinking it might be them."

The counselors were especially nervous, all sixty of them—roughly equal to the number of campers expected to arrive. They tried to busy themselves but couldn't help glancing up, looking over, hearing a noise, wanting to be the first to catch a glimpse of the yellow school buses. The majority of the counselors were young, in their late teens, but there were also parents among them—and even grandparents. They were there to serve, and they were beginning to see already that they would find out something about themselves before the week was out.

They also wondered, as did the others who waited anxiously with them, just how many of the children would actually come. They wondered if something might happen that week, something so terrible they'd have to call it all off, the whole effort, never to try again.

Each of them knew that many of the children they were going to meet would be experiencing an even more anxious "first time." For them, as Camp publicist Jack Slattery was to write, "being away from home usually meant a trip to the hospital—meeting a new person usually meant a new doctor or a new nurse."

Camp Good Days and Special Times was meant to change all that.

15

A Dream Gets Born

The sun reached high in the noonday sky and still no buses arrived. The counselors and staff sat down to lunch; it was quiet, almost eerily so. Then tough Lew Georgione, the waterfront director—old "leather lungs" they called him—thought he heard something. He blew on his whistle. He shouted that a bus was coming.

From every direction people came only to find that it was a false alarm—no bus or even anything resembling a bus. Georgione shrugged his shoulders and tried to look remorseful; Gary threatened to take his whistle away.

"They're here!" came a voice over the camp loudspeaker, and they came running, dropping everything, every inhibition. Some stumbled, some fell, but they got up again, running to the buses. It looked almost like the opening scene of "M*A*S*H," when the war wounded arrive.

They whooped and hollered, greeting that first bus from Rochester, surrounding it and pounding on its sides even before it had a chance to stop. They jumped up and down clapping and shouting "hello" as if they were meeting the most important people in the world.

For nearly 200 miles the children themselves had been giddy with excitement, shouting to each other and from the bus, but now they were silent. Small faces peered from inside the bus. They looked puzzled, unsure what all the excitement was about. Was it—could it possibly be for them?

Sande Macaluso watched, standing near Skip DeBiase. Both were tough men, growing up in tough city neighborhoods, but they couldn't stop the tears from falling now. Cheryl leaned against her husband, biting on her lip.

Muggs Register wanted to climb on board the bus and begin hugging the children. She wanted to get on with Camp without having to wade through all those awkward wasted moments of getting to know one another. She banged on the bus door until it opened and went inside while the kids were still in their seats. Polly Schwensen, watching Muggs, whispered a prayer that everything would be all right that week, that none of the children would get hurt or die.

Frank Towner, a college student dressed as a clown and named "Crossroads the Clown," blew long and hard on a blue horn. Though his face was reddened and it made an awful sound he kept blowing it anyway, like the angel Gabriel welcoming visitors to a new kind of heavenly kingdom.

For Sheri Mervis, the moment *was* just like heaven. She stood off to the side, with her family, away from the others. Teddi peered out from behind her mother, watching carefully as one by one the amazed, and seemingly dazed, children got off the bus. They looked like small soldiers on leave from a war.

Tod, naturally friendly like his dad, started shaking kids' hands and patting them on the back. He carried bags to cabins and came back again and again to carry more. Kim, the quiet Mervis who kept a lot inside, felt a terrible pain of recognition rise up inside her now. It would be one of the few times in her life she would remember feeling really upset. It bothered her that she had no way of knowing, before this, just how many children there were with cancer.

Dynamo Gary Mervis was still unable to fully absorb what was happening. The children had come, had taken a chance. And Gary Mervis, who is not demonstrative of his emotions under normal circumstances, began to cheer— for the children, and for all those who had helped, who had given, and who had prayed. Tears fell from his eyes, his wife beside him crying, too. Dreams could and did come true.

Laurie Allinger then came down the steps of the bus. All she could remember afterward was: "They were cheering so much I felt as though I was on top of the world. They made you know they were there to give you something—that you weren't going to be able to lay down and do nothing."

Laurie Kaleta, "Froggy," felt both scared and excited. She was anxious to meet Teddi, anxious to get on with the Camp, but she seemed overwhelmed by the emotion of the moment, seeing so many others who had gone through what she had gone through. It was such a clear break from the world she was normally in that it seemed intimidating at first. Along with the two Lauries, thirty other kids got off the bus, and the hands of staff and counselors kept reaching up—to help them, to greet them, to touch them.

The buses from Syracuse and Buffalo arrived within the hour, and these children, too, were greeted with the same intensity and enthusiasm as that first bus. Suzie Parker climbed down off the Syracuse bus, saying afterward: "There was nothing like it. Nothing in the world like it."

Before dinner that night, while they were all noisily together, the Camp had its first mail call. Many parents had written letters during the week so that they would be there when their kids arrived. Some parents were certain their children would be feeling homesick and a letter from home might help. Other parents wanted to stay connected to their children, despite the miles and time. One little boy received three letters from home in one day and the dining room crowd rose in one thundering, standing ovation upon hearing the announcement. Such applause and ovations were common at mealtimes during the week. Every small moment received spectacular attention.

At the first camp dinner, after everyone was seated, Gary Mervis was introduced. Campers, counselors, and staff rose to their feet again, clapping and cheering. They wanted to say thank you in a big way to the man who had made all this happen, who had brought them together and out of isolation. If ever there was an election for the campaigner, with a landslide victory, then this had to be it.

Gary slowly rose, waiting for the cheering to subside. He leaned on the table with his hand. His legs felt unsteady as he looked around the room. He took it all in, conscious of the moment and not himself, going from face to face of new people, children he had only seen pictures of, friends who had stood by him when the dream was new and the doubters many.

Gary would bring the house down that night with his promise to the kids that he would wear the same hat backwards, and wouldn't shave, as long as the sun kept shining. When it did finally rain, Gary shaved his scraggly beard, and the kids thought his hat deserved a proper burial. They took it down to the dock, filled it with rocks, and as the trumpeter played "Taps," tossed it out to sea.

Teddi still wanted to stay with her mother, in her mother's cabin, but Sheri didn't think it was a good idea. If Teddi was separated from the other children, even at night, she might never feel like she truly belonged there. Teddi would miss those late night talks when peers would get to know each other, share intimacies, perhaps even form bonds of friendship.

And this is exactly what happened that first night, inside the cabin that Teddi was in. Counselor Anne Kiefer was in charge; Laurie Allinger, "Froggy" Kaleta, and Suzie Parker were also in the same cabin. It didn't take long for the four of them to gravitate to one another, and to probe each other's own cancer story.

"Did you have radiation?" Teddi asked the three others.

They all nodded. Two of them had gotten real sick, too. Had Teddi?

"Not me," Teddi said. "But I did get awful tired—and my hair fell out!"

They looked at each other. There was a pause, then Laurie Allinger said her hair had fallen out, too. Suzie Parker said the same thing happened to her.

Teddi was warming up now. "Did you ever get to feeling at the hospital like you wanted somebody with you but you didn't too? Like you wanted them to hold your hand and not get bored, but not say anything either?"

They all talked about that, and about other things they had kept inside. Sometimes what they said was buried so deep they surprised themselves when they spoke the words. But not everything they feared and shared could be put into words.

"Next to saying good-bye," Laurie Allinger would recall, "the hardest thing for me at Camp was getting undressed that first night and maybe somebody seeing my scar." She didn't have to worry: everybody had their scars, some visible and some not.

Teddi, Laurie, Froggy, and Suzie quickly became friends. Laurie Allinger believed it was because none of them was really timid or shy, they all liked boys, and they all had the same attitude toward their cancer. "We're going to beat this thing," they would take turns promising each other, often in the dead of night, when fears are usually strongest.

They would all say afterward, all but Teddi, when they had time to sort the whole camping experience out, that Teddi was the "best" in the cabin, the sparkplug, their leader. "I got kind of down sometimes," said Allinger, the girl who would ride horseback and learn to water-ski with one arm, "and Teddi was always there and she would bring me up. If somebody felt kind of scared, Teddi would bring you out of it by saying, 'What's wrong?' She didn't seem scared of anything. She just came out and said, 'What's your name?' She was really outgoing."

Before the four of them did something especially different, like riding horseback or taking a plane ride, one of them might say to the others, "Well, I don't know. I'm kind of scared. I could get hurt." But Teddi would be there, and if not her, one of the others, lending encouragement. "C'mon," she could be expected to say, "we can do it! We've gone through tougher than this!"

Counselor Anne Kiefer recorded in her journal an incident that happened in the cabin one night.

One of the girls in the cabin sometimes had such severe pain she wanted her medication before the necessary time had elapsed. Anne knew it might be harmful if she gave the child the medicine, in spite of her pain. One night, as the girl rocked and moaned on her bed, Anne, pacing, found that Laurie was awake.

"Laurie," she said quietly, "have you ever hurt this bad?"

"You bet your bosoms!" the girl answered.

Anne smiled, wanting to know what Laurie did when the pain was this bad.

"I try to do something to take my mind off of it. You know, like watch TV or draw."

Anne took out colored marking pens and papers. Laurie, Anne, and the girl, working by flashlight, drew pictures and colored them until the pain pills could be administered. They continued to stay up a while longer, waiting for the girl's medication to take effect.

Sometimes, later in the week, the girl's groaning would take its toll on Laurie. It reminded her of what she had gone through, and what, in all likelihood, she would have to go through again. When moments containing these fears came, Laurie found herself leaning on friends Suzie, Froggie, and especially Teddi.

By mid-week, late one night, while everyone else slept, the four decided they wanted to be "blood sisters." No one afterward seemed to remember who came up with the idea, and maybe that's all just as well—for they all were eager to do it.

"Here. We'll burn a needle and then stick it in our finger," Teddi whispered—Teddi, the fireball instigator.

Suzie Parker got squeamish. "Well, I don't know," she shivered. "Why do we have to do that?"

"It's to seal our friendship," Laurie Allinger explained. "We do everything together, and we even talked about being like real sisters. Now come on guys, let's be blood sisters."

Suzie still hesitated, and Teddi took the needle and poked her own finger first. "Piece of cake," she said, "after all we've been through." She took Suzie's hand and steadied it, before poking the needle in her finger, too.

Then the four touched fingers, their blood mixing together. "All right," they exclaimed. "That does it."

A voice pleaded with them to be quiet. They giggled, and before turning in for the night, agreed on a toast. "To health and liberty," they said, together.

16

Good Days

Skip DeBiase had gone out to the dock alone that first evening. He needed to pull himself together from the emotion of the day. He stood there looking around him, admiring the sunset, the thick pines surrounding the lake, and the clear calm waters. He was still trying to think of something he could do that would be useful when it suddenly occurred to him that the one thing he knew well, and could teach the kids, was how to fish. Every kid, thought Skip, loved to fish.

Skip went to town for some bait only to be told that the lake was dead. Acid rain had killed it. There were no fish in the water, people said.

Skip drove back to Camp and went out to the dock again. He looked over the edge into the water. "It can't be," he said to himself. "It's too beautiful."

Skip drove into a different town, bought fishing poles and other gear. He found a kid selling worms and bought all he had, twenty dollars worth.

It was nightfall now, when Skip returned to Camp again. Others were in their cabins; he could hear people talking in the dining hall. He stood out on the dock by himself cutting up the worms and throwing the pieces into the water.

The next morning, after breakfast, Skip handed out fishing poles to the first dozen or so kids walking out of the dining room. Most of the kids had never held a fishing pole before. "Here," Skip said, sticking a pole into one hand and then another, "let's fish."

One of the adults stopped him. "You know the lake is dead, why do you want to get their hopes up?"

"It's sick yeah—but I don't believe it's dead," Skip answered.

Skip taught those who needed help how to bait the hooks. He taught them how to use a reel and cast. Those who had difficulty casting the line, he helped with taking hooks out of sneakers, and jeans, and the dock itself.

Their fishing lines were in the water for a few moments when the first child began shouting for Skip's help. He had a big one, the kid thought. It wasn't big, but it was a fish all right. A sunfish. And within a few minutes all the kids on the dock had caught a fish. Skip would cry every time a fish landed on the dock. One girl, one of the first to catch a fish that morning, was so excited and proud she kept the fish on a string in the water the whole week, making sure everyone at Camp had a chance to see it.

A typical day at Camp would include reveille at 7:00 A.M. This was immediately followed, for those who dared, by a "Polar Bear Swim." It was a suitable name, given the cold early morning Adirondack waters. Lew Georgione would notice that while only a few tried the swim early in the week, their numbers grew by the week's end.

There was a flag-raising ceremony at quarter to eight, followed by breakfast, then sick call and cabin clean-up. On any given day, children would spend an allotted amount of time at woodworking, arts and crafts, fishing, archery, boating, swimming, horseback riding, and playing at what were billed as "new games"—games which were fun but non-competitive. There was quiet time after lunch, and room for special events later in the afternoon. This was followed by dinner, a flag-lowering gathering, and night-time activities. Lights-out was set at 9:30 P.M.

Some things were typical for kids at any camp, cancer or not, such as writing home. Postcards, all written to Mom, were probably the same anywhere. One such postcard said: "Dear Mom, I miss you. I fell out of bed. I love you." Another child would write: "Dear Mom, Today I got E (a three backwards) letters. I went swimming. I didn't get tired on the way." And on still another postcard it was written: "Dear Mom: I am having fun. The first day we got here we went swimming. I like it here a lot. Nate." Then, in case his mother couldn't remember what her son looked like, Nate drew his picture at the bottom of his note.

Aside from the fact that there was a daily schedule of activities, and the kids wrote home just like they would at any other camp, hardly anything else at Camp Good Days and Special Times was typical. In fact, the Camp seemed every bit like the day set aside as "Backwards Day." On that day, people dressed backwards, walked backwards, and tried to do everything else backwards. "Backwards Day" was a good metaphor for the Camp itself, with dependent kids acting independent; kids who were "different" were not isolated and alone but now formed a small army of regulars.

Camp had its characters. Big Lew Georgione worked the kids hard in the water, trying to get them to learn how to swim. Sometimes the kids, legs kicking, would look up at Lew for a tidbit of recognition, a small crumb of approval. "I know I'm pretty!" Lew would growl back, "but pay attention to what you're doing!"

Another time, while checking cabins and tents one night, he poked his flashlight into Mike Menz's tent. "You awake, Mike?" he asked. Georgione never learned how to whisper, and Mike was startled. "Okay," Lew said, "you can go back to sleep now."

Late in the week, people decided that safety chief Sande Macaluso needed a night off. Usually he'd stay up through the night making sure the children, and others, would be safe. Nurse Mary Ellen Dasson and others told him to go into town for dinner, that they'd stay on guard.

It took some convincing but Sande went into town, along with lawyer Tom Gosdeck. When they returned, they were surprised to see nurse Dasson, obviously nervous, pacing back and forth in front of her cabin.

"What's the matter?" Sande asked.

"There's a bat inside my cabin."

"Okay," he said, "we'll take care of it. Be right back."

Tom and Sande went to their own cabin. Once the door was closed, Tom asked, "How the hell do you get rid of a bat, chief?"

"Damned if I know," Sande shot back.

They were laughing as they searched the cabin for something that might help them get rid of the bat. They found a ball of string and a broom, and took it back to where Dasson waited.

"What's the ball of string for?" she asked.

"I don't know," Sande said. "Maybe I'll lasso it!"

All of them were laughing now, and then Sande, Tom close behind him, crept up to the cabin door. Sande opened the door quickly and threw in the ball of string. "There," he said, after slamming the door shut.

Tom was confused. "What do we do now, chief?"

Sande looked at him non-plussed. "I did my part. Now it's up to you to do yours!"

In mid-week female counselors raided the men's cabins. It was partial payback for the night male counselors growled and scratched at their cabins pretending to be Adirondack bears. Next morning, over the Camp loudspeaker, came the messages: "Will somebody please return Judge Bonadio's shorts!" This was followed by: "Attention, Mary Ellen, we have your bat . . . "

Humor was an important part of Camp, and much of it had to do with Camp founder, Gary Mervis. He would ask one kid, for example, if he was having a good time.

The boy answered that he was.

"Let me know if you're not okay, Johnny," Mervis then said.

The kid nodded again. "I sure will, Mr. Mervis."

"Yeah, you let me know," Gary grinned, "and if you're not—I'll send you home."

Humor at Camp seemed a way to ease doubts, ease pain, and even change perspectives. At times, it seemed to give campers and counselors alike a kind of spiritual second wind. Humor was fundamental to courage.

Gutsy Laurie Allinger learned how to excel at archery that week even with one arm. She learned to hold the bow in her toes. Ricardo Venegas, from Syracuse, couldn't even hit the archery target that first day but at the end of the week walked off with the grand prize for excellence.

Mark Dillon, handsome, affable, was one of the best-liked kids at Camp. One of the local television stories broadcast about the Camp humorously depicted Mark missing swing after swing of softball pitches thrown him. Mark, a good athlete, smiled and never told the reporter about the rod recently put in his leg because he had broken it.

One of the special activities for the older kids at Camp was an overnight canoe trip to an island out on the Lake. The eleven-canoe expedition was turned back once because of a sudden, massive downpour. But when the rain subsided they set out again, and all of them made it to the island. Once there they gathered wood, made a fire to cook with, and pitched their tents. That night, after eating, they sang songs just like they did every night at Camp.

If the personal strength and camaraderie gained from this experience weren't enough, Bello Snyder told them later in the week that a group of his kids earlier in the summer, kids *without* cancer, couldn't make the strenuous trip in a canoe and he had to take them out to the island in a motor boat. Word of this got around Camp quickly, and everyone seemed to walk around with a measure more of pride.

Laurie Allinger, easily identifiable now not by her loss of an arm, but by the bandanna and mini–cowboy hat she loved to wear, spotted Dr. Klemperer standing on the beach looking out over the water. She came up beside him.

"Can I ask you a question?"

Klemperer turned. "Sure, Laurie."

"Doctor—is there going to be a camp next year?"

"I sure hope so," was his response.

"May I come?" asked the child.

Klemperer nodded. If there was proof that the medieval attitude of people toward children with cancer needed changing, she was standing beside him.

Syracuse's Jim Hajski, one of the tallest kids at camp, was also proof positive. Jim loved basketball and seemed to play it at Camp almost non-stop. He never talked much. He also wore a bandanna and hat to cover up his surgical scars. "It's nice to be out here," he said, "and not feel like a freak."

The people in Inlet, and around Fourth Lake, were slowly beginning to find out about Camp Good Days and Special Times, and the special children in their midst for a week. Out boating, or water skiing, they would make a special pass by the shore and blow kisses. Inlet's fire department came with its truck, sirens blaring and lights flashing, and took the children on a wild ride through country roads. A man who owned a custard stand gave free ice cream cones to each of the kids. "I saw their faces," he said afterward. "That was enough of a reward for me."

The kids thrilled at being able to go to the Enchanted Forest, or for a hike up a mountain trail. A large sightseeing boat took them around the Lake, a ski lift took them up mountains, they rode horses in the valleys, and an amphibious plane took batch after small batch of them soaring through the clouds.

Sheri thought Teddi was having the time of her life. Her nervousness about coming ended by the second day—she took off her hat and didn't care who saw her with no hair. The print and electronic media came to Camp and sought an interview with Teddi. Sheri thought her daughter answered reporters' questions like a "pro." Dr. Klemperer, watching the attention Teddi was getting, would say she did not act like "a reigning queen," that there was even "a modesty to her—a sense of humor and common sense that was really nice to see."

Though Teddi seemed to shed her nervousness all of a sudden, Sheri couldn't seem to let go of hers. In some cases she was more anxious than she might have been if Teddi were home. Sheri would check on Teddi at night to make sure she wasn't in any pain and to see that she was getting enough rest. She would give Teddi a kiss in the morning, at noontime, and before bed. This routine of affection did not go unnoticed by Teddi's "blood sisters" and the other girls in the cabin, who missed their moms. And so before long Sheri was kissing each of them morning, noon, and night. It helped ease some of the wound in Sheri's heart, and the worrying that plagued her mind.

Then, early one morning, as Sheri looked out over the Lake, she noticed Teddi going in for the Polar Bear Swim. At breakfast, Sheri asked Teddi what was going on—for she knew jumping into cold, cold water so early in the morning just wasn't Teddi's style.

"I've got a boyfriend," she told her mother, eyes beaming. "And he goes swimming in the morning." Teddi knew how protective Sheri felt. Teddi paused, leaned forward, and in a loud whisper told her mother: "I go so I can grab him!"

Early the next morning Sheri watched again, but this time Teddi stood on the shore, a blanket wrapped around her, watching. The third morning, Teddi didn't show up on the beach at all.

"What's the matter between you and Marvin?" Sheri asked.

"Nothing," Teddi answered nonchalantly. "He's interested in me without my going swimming."

Sheri laughed. "Good for you," she told her daughter. "Good for you."

Though Teddi went through nearly a half-dozen boyfriends during Camp, blond-haired, blue-eyed Marvin would remain special. Sheri was amazed at the boy's politeness. A year older than Teddi, Marvin would hold open doors for her. He politely asked her to the Camp's formal dance and held her hand that night. "Do you want some cookies, Teddi?" he'd say, and then he would go and get them for her.

The children at camp were divided into different cabins, which were named after Indian tribes. Boys and girls from the same tribe did many of the same activities together. One night, as Sheri was walking back from supper, she spotted Teddi ahead of her. She was walking with a boy, and it wasn't Marvin. When Sheri passed the same cabin that Teddi and the boy had just passed, she heard a voice from inside say: "We better get out there right away, men. One of those Oneidas is stealing our woman!"

Sheri looked around. Woman? There wasn't any woman around but her. Naw—she thought to herself, they couldn't be talking about my daughter. When the boys piled out of the cabin chasing after Teddi and the other boy she knew it was true. The next morning Teddi ran up to her, ecstatic with the news—"They're fighting over me, Mommy. Isn't it wonderful—the boys are fighting over me."

Counselor Anne Kiefer picked up a different side to Teddi that week, a side that may have gone unnoticed in the whirlwind of activity and attention. Toward the end of the week, Kiefer would write in her journal:

> . . . I sat next to Teddi, who was very quiet. I could think of nothing to say to draw her out that would not seem false or hypocritical, so I left her alone with her thoughts. I guess I could have teased her out of her mood, but sometimes teasing takes a nasty turn. She was already impressing me as being introspective, a little aloof, maybe even a little depressed.

Anne thought Teddi may have been somewhat envious of her sister Kim, who Anne described as "an exceptionally pretty thirteen-year-old." Though Teddi idolized Kim, self-consciousness about her own looks—despite the attention she was receiving from boys—may have had an effect. Anne also speculated that Teddi was having trouble separating her desire to be just another camper from the attention afforded her as being the Camp's inspiration.

As the week drew to a close, many began to sense how hard it was going to be to leave. It came out in odd ways those last few days: a boy suddenly stops talking to a girl he was trying so hard for so long to get close to; a girl suddenly bursts into tears because she made a mistake in passing the salt and not the pepper. It got harder and harder to sing a camp favorite, "Kumbaya." Words such as, "Someone's crying, Lord, Kumbaya—someone's crying, Lord, Kumbaya," at times made people stop—kids and the others—to catch their breath or brush away a tear before joining in again.

There were other songs, too, which broke the heart. Beautiful nine-year-old Jennifer Masters stood center stage on talent night and belted out the hit song from the musical "Annie." "Tomorrow! Tomorrow! I love you, tomorrow!" she sang, and no kid knew how much the word "tomorrow" meant than the kids joining in, singing the final chorus with her.

17

Special Times

Suzie Parker remembered they would stay up all night that last night at camp, would talk about all they had done, the boys they liked best. It was as though they wanted to get things right, the details and exact words spoken, recall it all for one last time and then take it home with them inside, like a great harvest, with winter at the door.

The next morning was chaotic and tense. Clothes had to be found, sorted, and put in the right camper's bag. Each camper had to be put on the right bus. And all this had to be done in time for the buses to leave. Parents at the other end of the bus ride would be worrying.

Suzie Parker hugged Teddi long and hard; tears ran down her cheeks. She even hugged Tod, too, that day, even though Tod had put rubber mice and a rubber snake inside her sleeping bag. And she hugged Gary Mervis as well, whom she said was like a father to her, like her own father. She called out to Sheri: "See you next year!"

Laurie Allinger didn't want to leave at all. It was hard for her to see the buses come. And she was crying when she said good-bye to Teddi. Though some people told her not to cry, Laurie looked around and it seemed that everybody else was crying, too.

They cried not only for what they were leaving, but also for what awaited them. At most camps, kids are sad because they may not see their friends for another year. At Camp Good Days and Special Times they knew that they or their friends could die before another year went by.

Teddi held onto her emotional self. "Don't hang onto 'good-bye,' " she told Laurie, "keep trying to say 'hello.' "

Teddi's words made Laurie cry even harder. "Here's Teddi again," thought Laurie, "just like always, trying to bring me up." And then she whispered in Teddi's ear: "It was the best time in my life."

Teddi started to cry, too, when Marvin boarded the Buffalo bus. She waved and kept blowing him kisses.

Sheri, watching, thought Teddi was getting carried away. "Teddi—slow down," she said, putting her arm around her. "Just what have you and Marvin been doing anyway?"

"We haven't been doing anything more than you and daddy," Teddi answered.

"And what's that?" Sheri asked nervously.

"You and daddy kiss and hold hands, don't you?"

Sheri nodded, her calm returning.

"Well, that's what we've been doing," Teddi added, turning and continuing to blow Marvin kisses. Then she stopped, looked up at her mother, "There's nothing dirty about kissing, is there?"

Sheri told her there wasn't. She blew a kiss to Marvin, too, though inside the experience of Teddi holding hands and kissing a boy was too new for her to fully deal with yet.

Gary drove home with Doug Brown. Together they analyzed the positives and negatives of what had happened and talked about what they might do differently the following year.

Sheri, Tod, Kim, and Teddi rode home together. Kim stared out of the window: she had had a great time, met some boys, made new girlfriends, and had become an "honorary" aunt to little Jenny Masters—the girl who had sung "Tomorrow." She had also initiated the "tuck in" ritual at Camp. Older kids tucked into bed the younger ones and gave them a goodnight kiss. On the way home Kim remembered feeling pretty "full."

While Tod slept, exhausted from the experience, Teddi wrote feverishly. Like most kids, she loved to get mail, and now she was writing letter after letter to all the new people she had met, including, and most especially, Marvin.

Sheri was pleased Teddi had made some new friendships; it was what she had wanted ever since that terrible night she let Kim go to Chrissy's house, leaving Teddi behind. It was wonderful, too, thought Sheri, that Teddi had gotten a boy's attention, that she had been able to experience the feeling of falling in love. She pictured Teddi blowing kisses to Marvin once again. This time, Sheri began to smile.

She recalled a recurring exchange with Teddi, and wondered if it would happen any more.

Teddi would invariably ask: "Mommy—am I going to be beautiful?"

"Well, Teddi," Sheri would say, "you're very cute."

"But I don't want to be cute," Teddi would complain. "I'd rather be beautiful. Kim is beautiful but I'm only cute."

"Yes, that's true," Sheri would answer, "but I think you're charming, too."

"But I want to be beautiful," would always be Teddi's closing line.

Maybe now, thought Sheri, Teddi would come to understand what she always felt was true, that it was Teddi's personality that made her especially beautiful. Teddi found that summer at camp that boys liked her, and people liked being around her, not because of what she looked like but for who she was. Her baldness and lack of a wig made that unequivocally clear.

Skip went down to the dock late that afternoon, the camp nearly empty now. Busy as always, Cheryl was attending to some last minute details when Skip told her, "Don't come to get me—I'll be back when I'm ready." Cheryl saw that his eyes were reddened.

Skip sat at the dock's edge by himself. He thought about that week, and about John Davis, a wisecracking, troubled kid from the inner city. They had had a rocky beginning but left as good friends. Memories of John made Skip laugh while tears fell.

John had put shaving cream in Skip's pillow, covered Skip with whip cream, and even bombed him with water balloons. One time, when he had taken a group of campers out to an island in his boat, they realized that John was missing. They searched all over. Skip found a couple picnicking and they said they hadn't seen the boy.

Just then Skip noticed that their picnic basket began to rise in the air. He followed the fishline to the fish pole he had given John Davis who was up in the tree using it to reel in the basket lunch.

Later, after camp was over, Skip would call John on the phone and they would talk. Sometimes he'd drive down and pick the boy up in his flashy yellow Corvette convertible and take him to lunch, or back to his house for dinner.

Skip had been so busy teaching the kids how to fish, baiting their hooks, and taking those same hooks out of the fish, sneakers, and dock, that he didn't spend as much time as he would have liked with Teddi. He did make her come out to the dock and fish sometimes, even though he was aware that she was more interested in boys than fishing.

"You know," he had told her, "the reason you're out on this dock with me is so I can keep you away from that kid. What's his name? Marvin? I see you two sneaking in the bushes. I better not catch you!"

And Teddi would blush.

"Hey," he'd continue, "what kind of a name is that anyway? Marvin. Is he Italian? Ask him if he knows how to make spaghetti. What are you going to do with a guy who doesn't even know how to make spaghetti?"

Still reminiscing, he flashed back to that afternoon in the hospital parking lot, when Gary was crying, and how he had to leave the hospital himself when Teddi came back from surgery. He looked at the water again. "They said you were dead but you weren't," he told the lake.

Skip got up from the dock. As he walked back to the campgrounds he wondered if Autumn would be a hard one on Teddi, and the kids at this special Camp. He hoped that each would carry the warmth of a special time well into winter.

Autumn was warm that year. Teddi went to school. She became a cheerleader for one of the Vince Lombardi teams; her father coached another team, a team Tod played on. They would kid each other at supper about which team was better, how terrible the referees were.

Despite the hectic pace of their lives, the Mervises tried to find time for their other children as well, straining to resist the natural tendency to give the majority of their attention to the child who needs it most. Still, they knew that when Teddi talked they seemed to listen a little harder than when Tod and Kim spoke, searching for the fuller implications of Teddi's words.

Teddi continued to stream out letters to some of the friends she had made at camp, to her "blood sisters," and to Marvin. In one letter she even invited him to come to Rochester to see her.

Sheri took the phone call late one Friday afternoon that Autumn. It was Marvin's mother. Her son was on the train to Rochester which was due to arrive at 7:30 P.M. Sheri told her that was fine, hung up the phone, and asked Teddi if there was something she would like to say to her. Teddi said she couldn't think of anything, and then Sheri reminded her about Marvin's visit. "Oh, I didn't think he'd really come," Teddi told her mother. Sheri shook her head saying, "It's a good thing we're going to be home this week-end."

Throughout that Autumn Teddi made suggestions to her dad about how to improve the camp. She continued to talk about her experiences at camp, what had happened, who said what to whom and why. She went over it, again and again, until it began to settle deeply inside, beyond touching but never beyond remembering.

Sheri would listen and smile and feel so hopeful that sometimes she couldn't believe Teddi was really sick at all. Her November check-up was encouraging, Dr. Salazar noting that Teddi was "doing very, very well." Her hair was growing back. Though she still had some lack of coordination in her left hand, she did not seem to favor it.

Yet despite these and other positive developments, the dark circles around Teddi's eyes persisted. Sometimes her eyes even looked glassy. There were seizures too. They never lasted long, but they wouldn't go away either.

Sheri found herself worrying about the oddest things, like the time Teddi had a sore throat and she worried if somehow it was related to the tumor. She worried when Teddi had novocaine at the dentist's office, or when the dentist took X-rays, knowing how much radiation Teddi had had already.

None of the doctors speculated about when the tumor might start growing again, or how much time Teddi had left. And neither Gary nor Sheri opened the door to such matters.

They took care of the doctor's appointments and got the required tests done on time. But other than that, they just watched and waited, wondering—as it were—when the other shoe would drop.

18

The Sound of the Second Shoe

It was a dreary, desolate January day when Teddi went with her dad to Dr. Salazar's office for still another CT scan. Afterward, after telling them both about the test results, he put his arm around Gary. Teddi had gone on ahead of the two now. "I don't want to get your hopes up," said the doctor, "but eighty percent of the recurrences take place within two years. In April it will be two years. If she makes it to then, she has a chance of making it."

But it wasn't long afterward that the number and seriousness of Teddi's seizures began to increase markedly. Sheri was alarmed. After consulting Dr. Nazarian, Teddi's pediatrician, Teddi's Decadron dosage was increased but it didn't help. "She's getting worse," she told Gary. "We should take her in to see the doctor."

Gary resisted the idea of taking Teddi in. He wanted April to come and go first. "She's the same as she always is," he would answer. "Let's not go looking for things."

Sheri let it go until she knew that something had to be done. "You've got to take her in," she pleaded. "Something's bothering her."

Dr. Salazar seemed troubled by the fact that Teddi's tongue, upon protusion, deviated significantly to the side. He asked for and received an immediate CT scan. Nelson came up to examine the results along with Salazar. They found a large cyst on the tumor but weren't sure if there was regrowth of the tumor itself. There was no way to be certain other than a repeat craniotomy.

Nelson was initially against the idea of more surgery. He felt it was too close in time to the previous operation. Salazar, on the other hand, thought re-radiation might be more successful if there was a second craniotomy. Gary listened carefully to what they were saying, his emotions numbed. Radiation had worked pretty well before; maybe combined with new surgery it would work again. "I have to ask Sheri first," he told them. "Could somebody call?"

He wanted to explain why but Teddi was there, eyes straight ahead, but listening, always listening.

It was four o'clock. "I think you better come down here," Salazar's assistant told Sheri.

Sheri sat with Gary, Teddi, and the two doctors. She could see how tense their faces looked. Gary told Sheri about the cyst and about the reasoning behind a second operation. Nelson explained that he would try to remove the cyst in a second re-entry into Teddi's head and get out as much of the adjacent tumor as possible. Salazar then said he would try localized radiation. Chemotherapy was also an additional therapy consideration.

Gary talked with Teddi and asked if she was willing to go through more surgery. Sheri watched Teddi as her husband talked. She was holding onto Teddietta tightly. Sheri put her fingers to her lips and for some reason nodded her head slowly up and down. She closed her eyes, not wanting to cry any more. When Gary was finished, Teddi told him if he thought it would help then she would do it.

Teddi was readmitted to Strong Memorial Hospital on January 18, 1981. The admitting physician's report said that Teddi was weak on her left side, that she couldn't raise her arm above shoulder length, and that there was poor use of the fingers on her left hand.

Upon admission, Teddi met up again with nurse Anne Cameron. Teddi had met Anne the first time she was admitted to the hospital. Anne had volunteered to take her on a tour of the pediatric floor and had talked about Teddi's first operation with her. Now Anne maneuvered to get Teddi placed on the pediatric floor rather than the adolescent floor. Her age now would normally put her on the latter, but Anne felt that the change would make it emotionally harder on Teddi, that she wouldn't know anybody and would have to meet—and come to trust—everybody all over again.

Anne had followed developments with respect to Teddi since their first meeting. Teddi had been written about in the newspapers, and Anne had seen her on television. Teddi was often seen laughing and appeared happy. But Anne knew not all of Teddi's tumor had been removed, and that her tumor was the kind that was deadly and would revive itself sooner or later.

Anne Cameron would assume "primary nursing care (PNC)" for Teddi. At Strong Memorial Hospital, one of the few hospitals featuring such care, PNC meant that one nurse was generally in charge of all aspects of a patient's care. Such an approach, it was felt, would give patients and families alike a sense that there was one primary contact person. This one person could come to know the patient and them well. Versed in the medical aspects of treatment, this person could also maintain some continuity between the new faces, nurses and doctors alike, that make hospital stays nerve-racking and worrisome.

There was, however, a big emotional risk for the primary care nurse. Such emotional intimacy was often harder to endure than the shift in, shift out approach. Relationships formed, making the pain a personal experience should the patient die. It would be like losing a friend over and over again.

Barb Fredette and Sally Masten would also become involved in Teddi's case, and with Teddi and her family. They would provide secondary nursing care. The introspective Barb Fredette, reflecting upon the pain involved in such emotional intimacy would also say that there was a lot of love involved in such relationships as well, and that if she had foregone the pain she would have missed the love, too.

After succeeding in the placement of Teddi on the pediatric floor, Anne went into Teddi's room and introduced herself to the Mervises, explaining what her role was and the floor routine. As she talked, she noticed and would remember afterward how utterly tired Sheri looked. Sheri seemed as though, thought Anne, she wanted the whole sorry business done with once and for all.

It was often difficult for primary care nurses, even ones as open and thoughtful as Anne, to get to know their children well in the beginning. Parents tended to speak for them at the outset. But Anne soon found quiet times to be with Teddi and together they built a strong and trusting nurse-patient relationship. This quickly turned into what seemed an older sister-younger sister bond.

Teddi told Anne about Teddietta, and how Teddietta had been with her since she was a baby. She told Anne about all the other teddy bears people had given her. She showed Anne a picture of her dog "Sweet'ums," too.

"Everybody says she's ugly but she isn't, do you think so Anne?"

Anne couldn't keep from laughing. "I'm sorry, Teddi," she said, looking at the picture again. "She really is ugly!"

Teddi laughed, too, later telling Anne about Marvin, and the boys at camp who had fought over her, the ones who still wrote to her and wanted her to write back. She told Anne about Skip's son, too, who always flirted with her—and how she sometimes flirted back, too. Anne and the other nurses would take great pleasure kidding Teddi about who her boyfriend for the day was.

Becoming close to Anne made a difference as the time for surgery approached. In the days immediately preceding surgery, Anne came in often even though some were her days off. She tried to choose the words she spoke to Teddi carefully, watching Teddi's face for any hint of fear and self-doubt, and would try to comfort her, sometimes by just holding her hand.

"The pre-operation shot is going to sting, Teddi," Anne explained.

"Why does it have to hurt?"

"Well, the doctor has to give you the shot in your thigh because they find that's the best place for children to absorb the medication to make you drowsy. That way you won't feel the pain later in surgery."

"They do that so I can go to sleep and not feel any pain, right?"

"That's right," Anne soothed.

"My dad told me. And I was in here before, so I kind of remember what it will be like."

"There'll be some pain after," Anne told her.

"I know, just like before. But after awhile I'll be all right," she said, turning her face away from Anne.

Anne went over the operation procedures with Teddi several times, explaining what they would do and how they would do it. She couched her words so as not to arouse new fears and tried to be directly responsive only to what Teddi truly wanted to know. She found that talking too much, and about what adults thought important, could be every bit as painful as a doctor's needle and a surgeon's scalpel.

The night before surgery, before her mother and father left, Teddi said she was afraid. She also said she wanted to have surgery done so she would be able to be well and feel good again. She asked if they would be there in the morning before she went in for surgery. They promised they would be there and kissed her good-night.

Next morning, Gary was running a little late. He kept forgetting things, like a man who subconsciously doesn't want a day known to be hard to begin. Sheri waited in the car, beginning to panic, blowing the horn. She needed to see Teddi before surgery, and as Gary sped to the the hospital she kept looking at her watch. Gary dropped her off at the front of the hospital, and went to park. Sheri rushed inside and found that Teddi had already been put on a table to be wheeled down to the operating room. She delayed the orderly, and some of the staff there, until Gary had a chance to get there.

Sheri didn't wish Teddi luck that morning. She told Teddi she would be there when Teddi came out. "I love you, honey," she told Teddi. Secretly, Sheri didn't think Teddi would survive surgery a second time. She didn't tell Gary this because she didn't want to add to his worry. But she had the same feeling she had had a few days before, when she knew the seizures were different from the seizures before, that terrible sense of foreboding special to a mother's heart.

Gary understood how serious the operation was going to be. He had taken medical books out of the Hospital library and studied the procedures. He had raised questions with both Salazar and Nelson. Still, he was trying to hang onto hope. "What if . . . ," he kept saying to himself, "What if it's just a cyst and not a regrowth and they're able to clean it all out. What if . . . ; what if . . . ," again and again.

Dr. Nelson entered the operating room. Teddi had been thoroughly anesthetized and was in a deep sleep. Her head had been turned to the right, exposing his previous incision. Nelson helped prep and then draped Teddi's head. Deftly, he reopened the old incision. He turned down the scalp flap, and then removed the sutures. This exposed the dura. Teddi's brain, to Nelson, seemed to be extremely—and it was his word—"tense." He opened and hinged the dura.

Nelson then saw the cyst and asked for a needle. He drew out approximately 22 CCs of a yellowish-looking fluid. Teddi's brain immediately went slack. The cyst had definitely increased pressure on it. The doctor probed further, to the tumor itself. He found it was yellow in color and covered with blood vessels. Its color and consistency told Nelson that the tumor had gone from an intermediate to a high-grade in terms of its malignancy. For the next several hours Nelson used suction to try and take out portions of the tumor. Several large arteries feeding into the tumor made suction difficult and dangerous. Doing as much as he could with suction, he then tried to remove still more of the tumor by actually cutting it out. The blood vessels bled quite vigorously with this approach and he did as much as he could without risking Teddi's life. He asked for a biopsy.

Nelson kept trying to remove pieces of the tumor. Though total resection wasn't feasible, he thought if he got out as much as he could it would ease pressure on Teddi's brain. By the looks of it, the tumor seemed as though it might continue to invade in the direction of Teddi's motor area.

Nelson straightened his back, which had become knotted and stiff. He looked at the clock. Nearly seven hours had elapsed. Having done as much as he could, he closed the dura with a silk suture, as he had done before, and then connected the craniotomy flap with #28 stainless steel wire. Nelson then sutured Teddi's exterior skin. It would have been quicker and easier to use staples, but they also carried the risk of infection.

As he was finishing, the biopsy report arrived. The tumor was high-grade, just as he had thought. It was further defined as a glioblastoma multiforme. Such rapid change in a tumor usually meant an extremely poor prognosis. He shook his head. He thought that Teddi would have twelve, maybe eighteen, months more to live. He didn't tell the others with him what the report said. He could tell by their faces that they knew; perhaps even knew what he was feeling inside.

Meanwhile, Polly Schwensen, the pediatric social worker at Strong who had challenged Dr. Royer when he visited Rochester and who had volunteered at that first Camp, sat with the Mervises while Teddi was in surgery. Polly remembered afterward that Gary would say this was the hardest time in his life.

Polly took Kim for a walk that morning. Later, she would do the same for Sande Macaluso and Judge Tony Bonadio. Both men were extremely shaken by how the Mervises looked; both couldn't believe Polly went through this time and again. They had come to know Polly at Camp. "Is this what you do? Is this it really?" they asked. "We had no idea."

Sheri sat in the special waiting room that Polly had helped obtain for her. It was private and only one family at a time could use it. Sheri knitted from the time she entered the room, seldom looking up. But after the sixth hour she broke down completely, sobbing and unable to stop. The others, Cheryl and Skip, Judge Bonadio, Irene, Bob Mervis, awkwardly groped for words of comfort. They tried to console by touching and stroking her, struggling all the while to control the emotional tornado lurching up inside each of them.

Sheri knew. Deep down she knew. She knew Dr. Nelson's findings were going to be bad but the waiting was unbearable.

When Dr. Nelson called that particular room, Sheri was still crying and shaking uncontrollably. All she wanted to know at this point was whether Teddi was still alive. It didn't matter if Nelson had removed all or even a little of the tumor. It didn't matter if Teddi had a day, a week, a year more to live. All that mattered to the mother now was whether she would see her daughter alive one last time.

Dr. Nelson, over the phone, said to Gary that he had taken out a grapefruit-sized tumor, but that there was still some left, and that it had threaded itself into other parts of Teddi's brain. He said he would be up to talk to them later.

"She's alive," Gary told his wife, holding her close to him now. Suddenly shaken by the fact that Nelson hadn't come up personally to tell them about the operation, he turned to a resident physician and asked why the doctor had not come.

The resident physician left the room and returned, moments later, with Nelson. The doctor explained again, though this time more briefly, what had taken place in the operating room. All the time he talked, Sheri sat there watching him. She felt overwhelming gratitude that Teddi hadn't died on the operating table. Yet some of the sorrow she felt was for the defeated look in the doctor's eyes.

19

Starting Over

"Do you know who you are and where you are?" nurse Cameron asked, her face close to Teddi's.

Teddi was once again in Strong's pediatric intensive care unit.

Teddi tried to open her eyes but they were swollen badly. "I'm Teddi," she managed, "and I'm at Strong."

"Good," Anne told her. She then told Teddi to rest and the child immediately fell asleep again. She slept fitfully that first night, and for the next few nights, becoming tearful at times because of the pain. The bandage on her head had to be replaced often, due to the bleeding, and this hurt her as well.

The Mervises told family and friends what had happened and was going to happen. The tumor was back again, they said, growing. Surgery had gotten a lot of it out but not all—it was too entangled with Teddi's brain. She would need radiation, maybe chemotherapy, and her situation would deteriorate. Difficult as it was to retell the story, repetition and the telling out loud seemed to help some, providing a kind of emotional relief.

Immediately after surgery, Polly noted in Teddi's chart that Gary "plans to do as he has done in the past, search for other medical answers." She also noted that "the family is obviously and understandably upset."

If these were hard days and nights for Sheri and Gary, and other adults in Teddi's life, it was all compounded for Teddi's siblings. It would take Tod and Kim many months, even years, to make sense of what was happening and be able to deal with their own fears and other emotions.

The day after surgery, February 13th, Teddi was taken out of the intensive care unit and put in a private room. She complained of headaches and abdominal pain. Her eyes were repeatedly checked for any deviations, just as they had been after her previous operation. The incision in Teddi's head, as was stated in her chart, seemed to be healing well. About four A.M. Sheri called the hospital to check on how Teddi was doing. Neither she nor her husband slept well.

Polly came by that day to discuss her role with the Mervises. Sheri spoke: "If you could stop by periodically, we'd like to talk to you about how we're doing. There'll be a lot we will be dealing with and maybe we could talk about that."

Polly wanted to know if they were generally satisfied with Teddi's care thus far.

The Mervises thought *this* admission had gone well. "We're able to relate to the doctors well and that feels good," said Gary. "Sheri and I both appreciate the openness and frankness of the doctors." The Mervises told Polly that they would like a straightforward, honest approach with respect to Teddi's care, and Polly passed this information on to the floor's medical personnel.

Teddi's eyes remained swollen, but she was capable of walking and did so, with help. She also got about with the use of a wheelchair. That night, after everyone had left, Teddi called Anne into the room. "I think I'm having a seizure," she said. "Will you hold my hand?"

Anne sat down beside her.

"I'm not always sure whether a seizure is just ending, or starting."

"Does that scare you?" Anne asked.

Teddi tried to nod her head, but it hurt too much. "Yeah," she said softly, "I can't control my arm."

Anne squeezed her hand, and began to stroke Teddi's arm. "I'll stay until it passes."

And so the two of them waited, quietly, in the darkened room whose walls were covered with get well cards, and spaces filled with potted plants and flowers. The eyes of bears and other stuffed animals, which were arriving almost by the hour, watched intently. The sound of Teddi's breathing told Anne the child was asleep. She bent down, kissed Teddi softly on the cheek, and tiptoed from the room.

The next day, the 14th, Teddi made an obvious breakthrough of sorts. The swelling around her eyes had gone down considerably, and she felt alert and energetic. The change put everyone in good spirits, including her father. "If you told me she would look this good a week ago," Gary told Anne, "I would have thought you were crazy." More for himself than for others, Gary then exclaimed: "I'm feeling really good now!"

Then Dr. Nelson brought up a CT scan done on Teddi. "It shows," he told Gary and Sheri, "that there's about a 70% reduction in the mass effect. Unfortunately, the scan also clearly shows plenty of residual tumor on all margins of the resection. It's my judgment she'll still be needing ancillary therapy."

Because Teddi again had to have radiation therapy, she knew the operation had not gone all that well. "They didn't get it all, did they, Mommy?"

"No," answered her mother, "they had to leave some fringes."

"Will they do anything besides radiation?"

Sheri said she didn't think so.

Later that day Gary met with Drs. Nelson and Salazar to talk about re-radiation of Teddi. Gary said he wanted to explore the possibility of chemotherapy as well. Chemotherapy involved the use of drugs. The particular drug, they agreed, would have to conform with the nature and location of Teddi's tumor. It would also have to be a drug with some proven success in terms of a glioblastoma multiforme tumor in children.

The medical record being kept on Teddi had grown long. Now they were starting volume two. The record contained medical terms, prescriptions, and hospital shorthand difficult for the layperson to understand; they are also devoid of humanistic insights and disclosures. Intended to be a technical record, entries seldom varied too far astray.

The days, months, and years, written numerically and separated by slashes, begin to stand out, making one long for the look and feel of the word "November" or "December." But on that day, February 14, another nurse entered Teddi's life. From the medical record, it was plain she would be different. In Teddi's chart that day, Valentine's Day, nurse Sally Masten had drawn a tiny heart.

From February 15 until Teddi was discharged on the 18th, she showed remarkable improvement. She slept well at night and was alert each day. Her spirits were good. Despite sustained weakness in her left hand, and several brief episodes of hand twitching, Teddi's wound healed well and she looked forward to going home.

Polly Schwensen observed in her official notes that Teddi had many visitors, including her aunt, grandparents, friends, and siblings. "Tod and Kim worked with Teddi on a puzzle. Then they watched TV. People took turns reading Teddi jokes from the newspaper." Polly also noted that Teddi's "dad was in good spirits," and that he had been doing extensive speaking on behalf of the Camp.

Before Teddi was discharged, the Mervises, in conference with Dr. Salazar, developed a re-radiation plan for Teddi. Radiation was to begin the following Monday, and she was to receive 150 rads per day for 5 ½ weeks for a total of 4,050 rads. Teddi's entire right upper brain quadrant was to be radiated.

It was impossible for Teddi to return to school after surgery. Her re-radiation therapy was to begin, and it was to be combined, at a later date, with some form of chemotherapy. She would need a tutor.

The Pittsford School District called Mrs. Karen Lenio, certified to tutor grades 1 through 6, and told her that they had a sick child who was in need of her services.

"What's wrong with her?" Karen asked.

"She has a brain tumor," came the reply.

Karen Lenio, a patient woman with children of her own, accepted the assignment, and after making arrangements with Sheri, drove over to see Teddi and meet the family.

Though it didn't show, Karen was nervous with each new tutorial assignment. Though having a great deal of experience, she always wondered if with each new time she and the family would be able to get along and feel comfortable around one another. She thought it a privilege to be invited into someone's home, and a considerable responsibility to be the sole provider of a child's education.

Karen Lenio didn't know what to expect either. Would Teddi be withdrawn? Would she be apprehensive about having a visitor, especially a teacher? What would Teddi look like? Would she have scars or be deformed in any way—handicapped perhaps? The official at the school district said he didn't know. Karen also wondered if Teddi would be able to learn at all, whether she would be able to keep up with her class and advance into 7th grade.

The afternoon Karen arrived, Teddi and Kim were on the couch watching their favorite show, "General Hospital." They laughed and agreed that Karen could have picked a better time to come. Though neither of the children noticed, nor the Mervises when they met her, Karen was deeply relieved. The family was friendly, and Teddi didn't seem at all embarrassed by her baldness, or the fact that she didn't have her wig on. "She's a pretty child," thought Karen, "and a spunky one."

Teddi, along with her parents and Karen, decided on a teaching schedule which consisted of one and one-half hours per day on Monday and Wednesday, and two hours on Friday. Immediately upon commencing, Karen was genuinely impressed by Teddi's commitment as a student. She accepted her homework assignments without complaint, always did them on time, and often asked for extra work to do. Karen decided she would try to keep Teddi up with her class.

From then until the end of March, Teddi also began re-radiation treatments. Dr. Salazar would note, toward the end of those treatments, that Teddi continued to have weakness in her left arm and left hand. He also showed Gary and Sheri a new CT scan which indicated there was a decrease in her tumor and the swelling around the tumor, compared with a CT scan taken prior to the initial re-radiation.

Salazar noted, in a March 31 report, that a meeting was being set up with Dr. Klemperer to decide which kind of chemotherapy Teddi would need. Even though the radiation treatment had been intensive, some of the tumor still remained. Salazar recommended chemotherapy as a way of killing it entirely.

A new, largely experimental drug called Cis-platinum was being tested at Georgetown Medical Center. It showed some promise in the treatment of tumors in children, and Gary had been following its developments with interest and care.

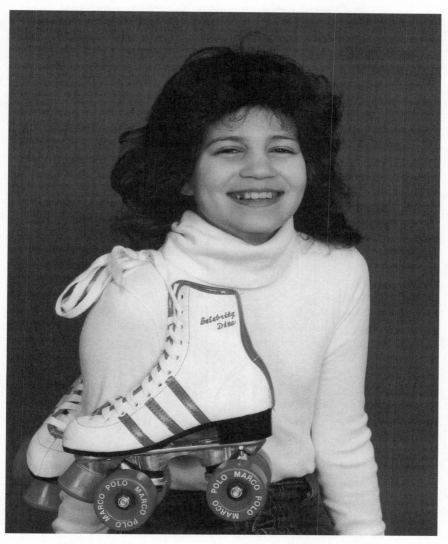

1. Teddi Mervis, a vibrant, active child, even in remission. Photo by Tony Pierleoni.

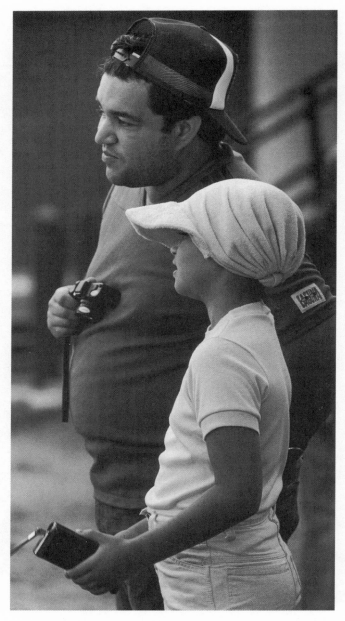

2. Gary and Teddi Mervis at Camp Eagle Cove in 1980. Photo by Dick
Sroda.

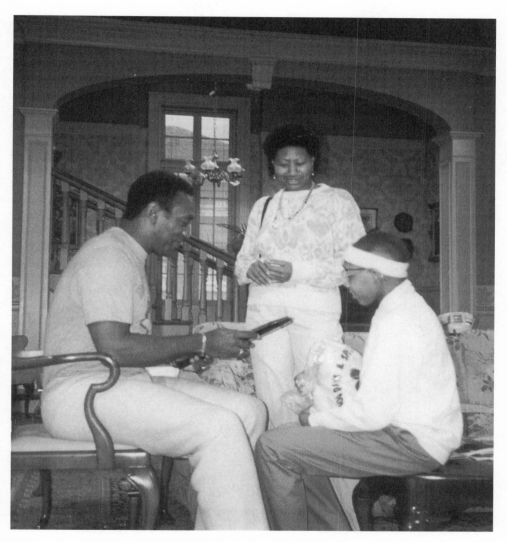

3. Clarence "Huggy" Pettway had a special wish and that was to meet Bill Cosby. Through the efforts of the Teddi Project that wish was fulfilled. Huggy's mother, Mary Pettway, watches as the two form what became a very special friendship. Photo by Tod Mervis.

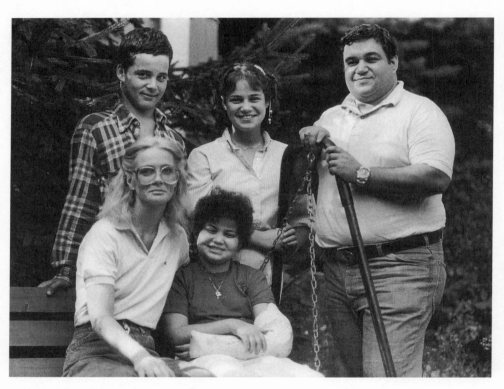

4. Teddi, shortly after her baptism, with her family. Photo by Kevin Higley.

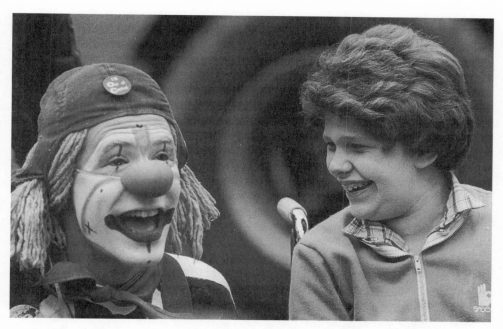

5. "Crossroads the Clown," one of the Camp's heroes, poses for a photograph with a young friend. Photo by Tony Pierleoni.

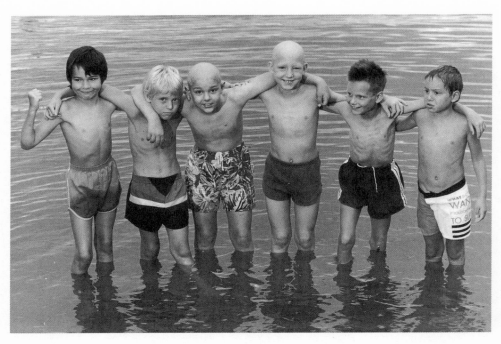

6. Six young campers pose for a photograph at the waterfront. Photo by Stephen D. Cannerelli.

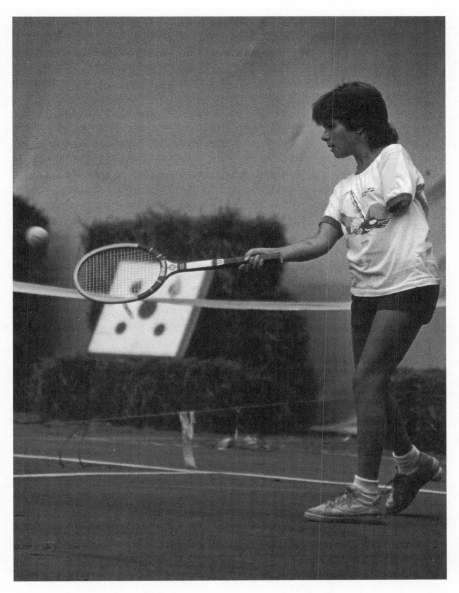

7. Disabilities resulting from cancer seldom deter campers from participating in the many sports activities being offered. Photo by Neal Haddad.

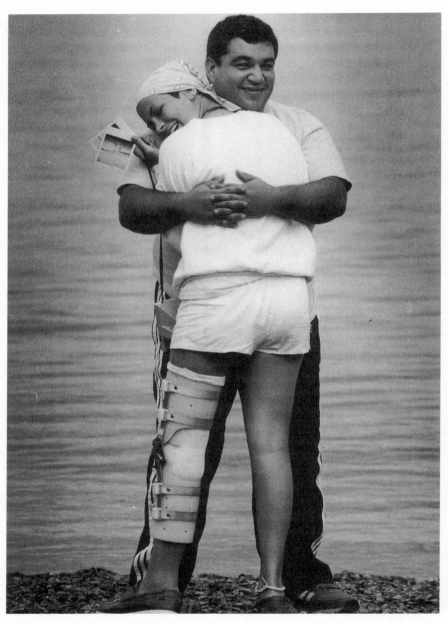

8. Gary Mervis, Camp Founder, shares in the memory of a previous summer with a returning camper. Photo by Neal Haddad.

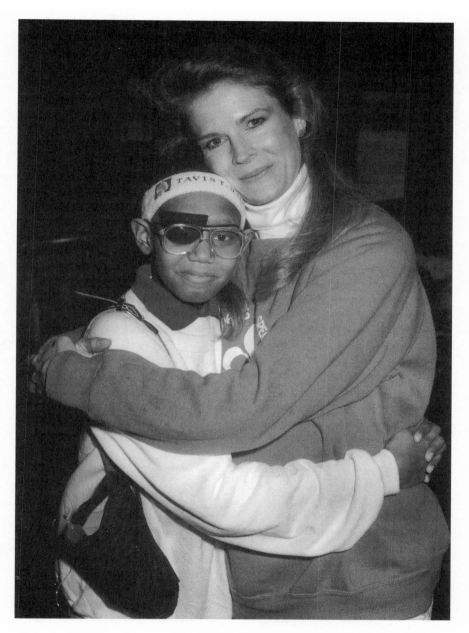

9. Candice Bergen and Clarence "Huggy" Pettway. Photo from the Camp Good Days' collection.

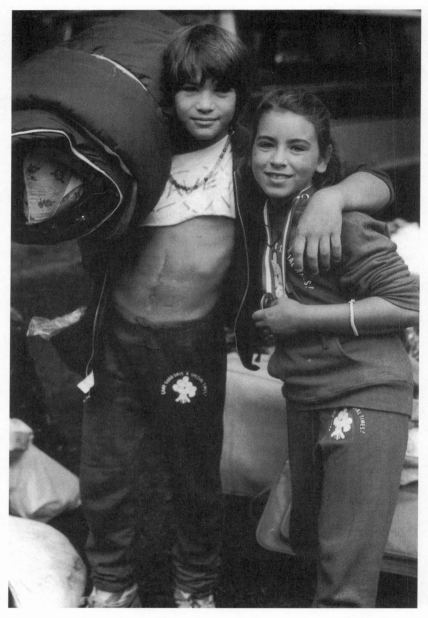

10. Getting ready to leave after becoming special friends. Photo by Neal Haddad.

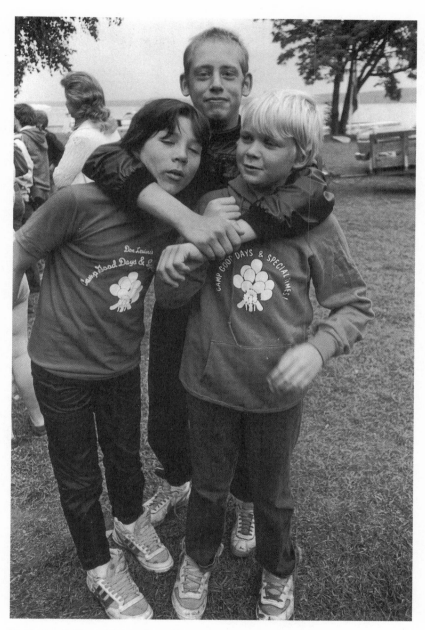

11. Saying hello at Camp after a long winter. Photo from the Camp Good Days' collection.

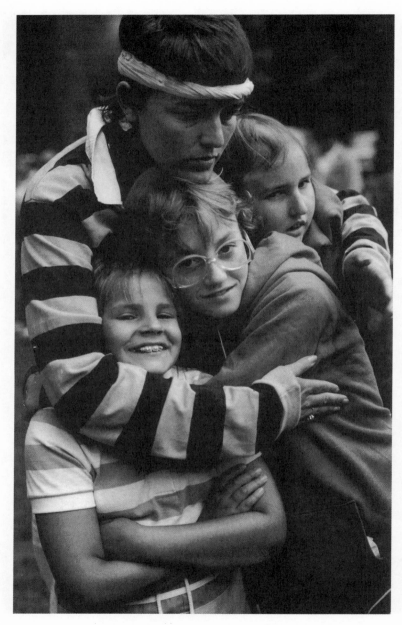

12. Saying goodbye after a fun-filled week at Camp. Photo by Neal Haddad.

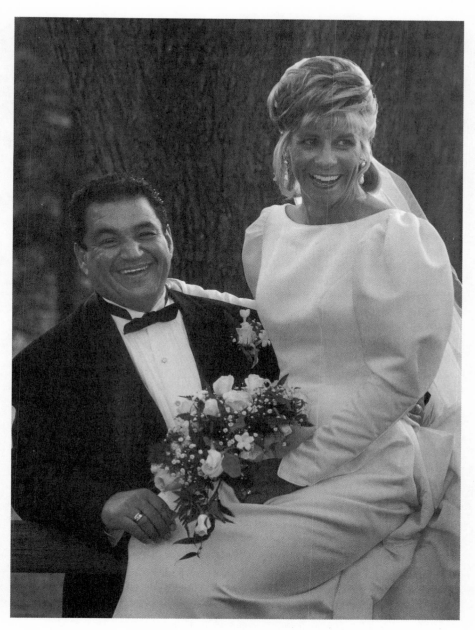

13. Gary and Wendy Mervis on their wedding day, June 10, 1995. Photo by Kevin Higley.

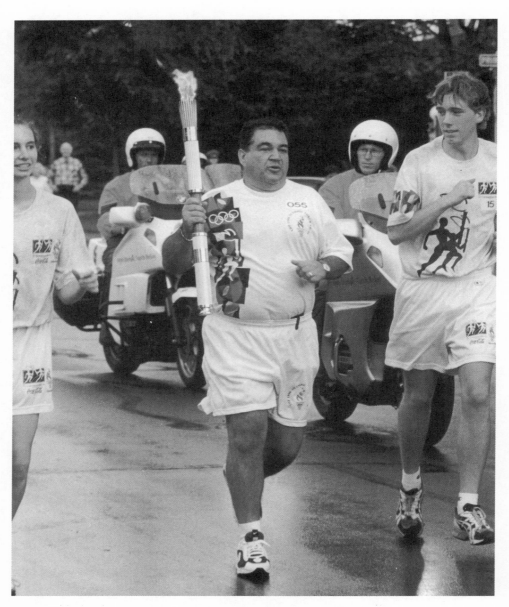

14. Gary Mervis carries the Olympic torch in 1996. Photo by Jenny Trynkus.

20

"I Love You Anyway"

Gary viewed the next stage of Teddi's treatment with cautious optimism. He asked Dr. Klemperer if he would take charge of chemotherapy treatment for Teddi. The Mervises trusted him. They had spent time with him at Camp, watched him with children, and listened to his views on how children with cancer ought to be treated.

Klemperer never let on, but one of the areas in human anatomy which troubled him most was the disease and treatment of the brain. He believed the mind separated humans from all living life, and to jeopardize its full function, or to lose that faculty altogether, caused him considerable anxiety.

"Yes, I'll do it," he conceded to Gary. Teddi and Sheri, who were also present, were as glad as they could be under the circumstances with his decision. Klemperer also said that he agreed with Gary that Cis-platinum was the most effective form of chemotherapy for children with a brain tumor.

"Cis-platinum does have nasty side effects," said the doctor, who believed in being honest with patients and their families. "In addition to nausea and vomiting, Teddi may lose her hearing. Her kidneys could also be permanently damaged." He stressed to them that there was no guarantee with Cis-platinum, even after enduring all its harsh side effects, that the tumor's growth could be halted, either briefly or altogether.

That afternoon, the four of them agreed they would proceed with Cis-platinum treatment until there was evidence that the tumor was growing again. If growth resumed, it would mean that the drug wasn't working, and the administration of it would cease immediately. Moreover, if the drug or its consequences proved too difficult for Teddi, termination would also be considered.

During the conversation that afternoon, Dr. Klemperer deliberately used the words "dying" and "death" instead of beating around the bush, holding out false hope, or using euphemisms such as "passing on" or "leaving."

Klemperer thought such unrelieved honesty, hard as it was at the outset, was the only way to emotional honesty and healing.

A little more than a month elapsed before Teddi began her chemotherapy treatments. Anne Cameron had talked to Teddi about Cis-platinum's effects on another child that Teddi knew. LaVerne Haley had been to Camp the previous summer. Anne knew LaVerne suffered from extreme nausea and vomiting.

Before Cis-platinum was administered, other procedures had to be initiated. Teddi was, for example, given the first of many I.V.s containing medicine to help prevent nausea and vomiting. Another I.V. was given to her to make her sleep during the ordeal of taking the drug. The night before treatment began she was hydrated. Right before the treatments began, Teddi would say to her mother, with no one else in the room, "Either you get better or you die." Then she turned to Sheri: "I'm not getting better, am I?"

"Honey, we're still trying. There's always hope and we keep looking. You've had two major operations and it takes a lot out of you."

"I'm not doing good, Mommy. I'm not well."

The following morning, and for nearly two days, Cis-platinum went into Teddi slowly, drop by drop, from still another I.V. inserted in one of her veins. Gary and Sheri were pleased, after the first day of treatment, because there were no adverse reactions to the drug, no nausea or vomiting, though they did express concern that Teddi acted a little disoriented.

After the second day of treatment was over, and after her parents and other visitors left the room, Nurse Barb Fredette went into Teddi's room to check on her and found her crying. Teddi didn't cry often. She was sensitive to how she hurt others, especially her parents, when she cried or complained. If a nurse was in the room when she cried, she would make them promise not to tell her parents, and in most instances the nurses complied.

To Barb Fredette, Teddi seemed to be the kind of person who kept a lot of her personal feelings inside. Though Teddi had a smile when there was company, alone she was more subdued and reflective.

"What's the matter," Barb asked, hoping she could be of help.

Teddi said she didn't want to bother Barb.

"You're not a bother to me," Barb said, taking Teddi's hand. "I'm interested in knowing what's wrong so I can help you."

There was a pause. "I'm afraid," Teddi said. She didn't look at Barb, instead kept staring at the ceiling. "I don't like being sick, Barb," she said finally.

Barb let a few moments pass before she asked Teddi what she was afraid of.

"Everything," was Teddi's answer.

Barb waited, trusting that patience was better than probing. Children often showed more faith in silence than adults.

Teddi then unraveled her fears, moving swiftly to the point. While she thought her sister and brother, and all her friends would be all right, she said she was worried about her parents. She was worried she was going to hurt them.

Barb wasn't sure what Teddi meant but Teddi seemed to be turning inward, so Barb let her go, believing there would be another time, that the heart of a child lets things out in trickles rather than a flood. Teddi's hand relaxed in Barb's and then fell to the bed as she drifted into sleep. Barb remained in the room for a few moments more, until she had regained her composure and could approach the next patient with cheerfulness and vulnerability.

Barb Fredette, like Sally Masten, knew Teddi's primary nurse Anne Cameron well. They had all been classmates at D'Youville College in Buffalo. Though Anne took her assignment in stride, both Barb and Sally weren't sure if they were ever going to warm up to the Mervises. Both were Teddi's secondary care nurses, Sally coming on board when another nurse voluntarily withdrew from Teddi's case. Sally described the Mervises, and especially Gary, as a "challenge."

Sally's view of Teddi matched Barb's more than it did most others. She didn't see the "corker" that her parents and friends described. For her, Teddi was a shy, mostly withdrawn child who preferred to stay in her room rather than wander the hallways meeting up with people, or going into the playroom to be with other children. She not only saw a child in considerable physical pain, but emotional pain as well.

Teddi had what is called four "courses" of Cis-platinum, beginning in May and ending in mid-July. Her second "course," in late May, resulted in serious new developments. Sally Masten reported that Teddi's seizures had changed, and were more strange and serious than before. Sally also noted that Teddi was losing the hearing in her inner ear.

With her third "course," and in spite of the fact that a repeat CT scan showed that the tumor was "much less prominent," Teddi's physical condition had deteriorated with terrible speed. Her suture now looked discolored, the scalp itself becoming "more tense." The medication forced Teddi to talk oddly at times, like someone who is disoriented. Sudden and sometimes violent muscular contractions occurred with regard to her left leg.

The Cis-platinum had taken a serious toll by mid-July, with her final course. Teddi was often nauseated and vomited frequently. Her face became disfigured, and she complained about her inability to sleep. She was no longer able to walk unless someone assisted her, and at home she stayed in bed most of the time. According to her medical record, Teddi could no longer hear the ticking of a watch or whisper. What wasn't in the record, but on everybody's minds, was the awareness that these changes signified the rebirth and growth of the deadly tumor again.

Though Teddi's physical condition declined throughout Teddi's treatments, Barb Fredette remembered her courage. "Most of us could go through chemotherapy the first time," she said, "but it's hard to come back knowing what it's going to be like. Teddi came in for treatment, that determined look on her face, and she took it time and time again—like a brave little trooper."

Everybody was feeling miserable at this point, including the doctors. Cis-platinum had resulted in blown veins for Teddi, the increased Decadron dosage had caused her to put on a great deal of weight. The result was that doctors couldn't find a vein in which to stick the I.V. needle.

Strong Memorial Hospital's policy is that a doctor had only three tries to get an I.V. in, then he or she would have to let someone else try. "Three times and you're out!" Barb remembered Teddi saying, trying to make the doctors feel better.

There were times when Teddi's own courage seemed to falter. Anne Cameron remembered how painful it was for Teddi to step on the scales with each hospital admission. With her last Cis-platinum treatment Teddi had stepped on the scale, watched Anne move the weight further and further to the right, and had blurted out: "I'm fat and I'm ugly, aren't I?"

No one present could answer or respond.

Sally Masten thought that Teddi was becoming increasingly frightened now, especially as the seizures came more frequently and with more violence. The medication and fatigue were making her terribly disoriented and this frightened the child too—Teddi was unable to determine if a seizure was just beginning or about to end. Anne and Barb noticed how increasingly withdrawn she had become. All Teddi's chatter about her boyfriends, and about Marvin, ended now, as did the nurses' teasing. Conversations slipped into phrases, and phrases gradually moved to one word questions and responses.

The nature of primary and secondary care nursing allowed Anne, Barb, and Sally to see and experience Teddi's deterioration intimately and up close. It was beginning to take an emotional toll on the three of them, and they tried to comfort one another when the nights were long and the courage thin.

After Teddi's fourth and last treatment, the doctor noted that while the Cis-platinum had apparently decreased the size of Teddi's tumor, the swelling around the brain had increased.

In his report the doctor also noted:

> . . . Teddy's (sic) father tells me that she knows she has cancer, a serious disease, but the family has not specifically dealt with death with Teddy (sic). The Mervises prefer to maintain an optimistic approach while she is undergoing her difficult treatments and wish not to dwell on the subject of death, saving all her energy for her treatments.

While a patient at Strong Memorial Hospital would have primary and secondary nursing care from the same people, physicians were a different matter. In Teddi's case, Drs. Nelson, Salazar, and pediatrician Lawrence

Nazarian would be her key consulting physicians but because Strong was a teaching hospital, attending physicians rotated.

The purpose of having "resident physicians" rotate was so they would gain experience on different floors, even different sections of the hospital, with different kinds of injuries, illnesses, and diseases. The drawback was that patients and their families sometimes felt intruded upon by strangers and lacked confidence with every new resident as to whether he or she really understood the patient's medical past and would make a mistake. It was an emotional burden on patient and family alike: They had to be more vigilant in monitoring patient care; they had to invest emotional energy in trying to get a bead on the new doctor in their lives.

These rotating physicians entered words into Teddi's medical record that others, close to her and the Mervises, never used. They often misspelled "Teddi," using a "y" instead of an "i" at its end. One doctor would write that Teddi was "obese." Another was touched by Teddi's circumstance. "It should be pointed out," he wrote, "that a grade IV astrocytoma's peak incident is 45–50 and is rare below the age of 30, making Teddy's (sic) plight all the sadder."

Teddi's recognition of her own seriousness, and her desire to explore this with her mother, came out when the Cis-platinum treatments ended.

"I'm going to be sick again, aren't I?" Teddi said, struggling to find accuracy in her words.

"Oh, Teddi," said her mother, "you know I wouldn't let anything bad happen to you."

But then Teddi said: "You know that's not true. You know you can't get rid of this cancer."

Sheri didn't say anything, nor could she move.

Teddi, noticing, went over to stand by her. Sheri was trembling now, ever so slightly. Teddi stroked her mother's arm, much like she did with her teddy bears, or a child would do with a kitten.

"That's all right," Teddi told her mother. "I love you anyway."

21

Decline

Teddi and her mother were at Skip DeBiase's house that spring visiting. At one point, Teddi asked if Skip would put a movie in the VCR for her.

"I've got just the perfect movie for you," he said, and put on "The Muppet Movie." He began to walk out of the room when Teddi called him back.

"Come here and listen for a minute," she said. "I learned the words to this song in school."

Skip knew the "Rainbow Connection," too, and knelt beside Teddi and started singing. The words, he said later, hit him like a train.

"Have you been half-asleep," they sang together, "and have you heard voices? I've heard them calling my name. Is it the sweet sound that calls the young sailor? The voice might be one and the same."

Skip began to cry, finding new meaning in the words, and feeling Teddi was trying to get him to understand and accept that she was going to die. He got up after the song was over and left the house. Sheri thought it strange that he left without saying good-bye, and that maybe he was mad about something, but Skip could never bring himself to tell her what had happened. After that time, and at different moments, Teddi would talk to Skip more and more about "not being around anymore."

Teddi talked to Cheryl, Skip's wife, about these things as well. One time she was telling Cheryl how great she thought heaven would be. Cheryl wasn't sure what she meant.

"Because I'll be pretty again," Teddi said. "I'm going to have all the boys I want. My hair is going to grow back. And I'm going to be *so* happy."

In some ways the campaign to raise funds for the Camp's second year was a little easier. At least Gary didn't have so much explaining to do about who he was or what the Camp was about. Many had heard of him and of the work he was trying to do on behalf of children with cancer by now. The Camp's first year had been an unmitigated success and word of that had gotten around as well. But foremost in the struggle to secure financial support, and ensure an ample supply of dedicated volunteers, was the fact that the Camp was not a dream any longer but a warm fact of life.

The high hopes regarding Teddi's schooling continued to erode. Karen Lenio still came to the Mervis home, and Teddi kept trying but returning to school was out of the question.

It hurt. Teddi wanted to go into the seventh grade very badly. It would have meant a change of schools: a different location with nobody else younger. There were horror stories which Teddi passed on to Mrs. Lenio, stories about seventh graders being shut away in their lockers all year.

That spring, before the end of the term, the elementary school Teddi would have normally been attending arranged a visit for sixth graders to their new school. There would be an orientation program as well as a chance to meet some of the "older" students. Teddy had looked forward to going. It was something neighborhood friends Tina and Jenny fervently talked about.

But when the time came for the bus trip from one school to another, Teddi wasn't able to go. She had kept up with her homework, sometimes refusing to sleep or to rest in order to keep up. But physically it would've been too hard on her; she just wasn't able anymore.

Sheri planned a party for Teddi on her birthday, June 27th. One of the people invited was Teddi's Camp "blood sister" Laurie Allinger. The invitation Laurie received said there would be pizza and that they'd all go out to a movie afterward. She called Sheri to say she would be coming.

Laurie arrived and was shown to Teddi's room. She looked around and Teddi explained there were exactly 187 bears and other stuffed animals in the room. Laurie's gift was still another small bear, wrapped in a shoebox. Laurie felt embarrassed, but mostly it was a deep sadness which began to fill her. Laurie's mother had told her that Teddi was not doing very well but the girl didn't pay attention—or didn't believe it was as bad as her mother was making it out to be. But there was no denying what she saw now. Laurie held back her tears as she helped Teddi open her present. She cried afterward though, while eating her cake at the far end of the table.

It was a hard summer for Kim. An active thirteen-year-old, she looked forward to being with her friends. Kim, along with Sheri, took major responsibility for Teddi's personal care. Kim washed her sister that summer, read to her, helped her to the bathroom and back. She was Teddi's steady companion. Later, Kim would feel bad about having become irritated with Teddi, frustrated by her demands or with feelings of being tied down.

Sheri would also have a hard time of it that summer. Teddi asked more questions. Sheri thought Teddi was afraid of the word cancer, and so she would say instead, when Teddi asked: "You have a brain tumor, honey." Though she knew she was softening the truth, she also felt that Teddi could not be at a Camp for children with cancer and not know. Teddi probably did know, knowing as well that her mother didn't want to talk about her dying. Teddi would say, maybe five or six times that summer, "Mommy, am I going to die?"

And Sheri would answer: "Teddi—we all die. We don't know when but it's going to happen."

On a few occasions Teddi said: "I certainly hope I die before you, Mommy."

Sheri told her that she hoped that wouldn't happen, that she couldn't live without Teddi.

"Well, Mommy," Teddi added, "I don't want to live without you either, so I'm just going to have to go before you."

Sheri continued to work at her day job that summer. She and Gary agreed that if Sheri provided Teddi with twenty-four hour care it might take too much out of her and even strain their mother-daughter relationship. Spending some time away, though it was hard for Sheri emotionally, seemed the best route to take.

It was, however, a physical strain. Not wanting to tie up precious time with extended grocery shopping, Sheri would stop home briefly after work to see Teddi, then run to the store for what they needed. This approach irritated Teddi at times. "I've been waiting for you all day," she said once, "and now you're going to get up and go and leave me?"

The Mervises bought a van so Teddi could go shopping with her mother and otherwise be able to be transported more easily. Still, it was an effort to get Teddi ready. She walked very slowly and so a half-hour run to the grocery store for Sheri, now took more like an hour.

One day, as Teddi waited in the front seat, Sheri, in getting the wheelchair out of the back of the van lost control of it. It began to roll on its own accord and Sheri fell, banging her knee, trying to stop it. Teddi watched, unable to help. After that she steadfastly refused to go with her mother again.

"I'm a klutz," Sheri told her daughter. "It wasn't your fault." But Teddi refused to go anymore anyway.

At the outset of her Cis-platinum treatments at Strong, Teddi talked to Anne about Camp, and about what a great time she had had the year before. She said she was really looking forward to going again.

But as Teddi's condition worsened, she talked less and less about going at all. In fact, as the date for Camp's opening approached, Teddi told her mother she didn't want to go. "I'm ugly, and I can't do anything anyway," she said. She was losing her hearing and it was clear to her that she was no longer able to take care of herself. A new test also disclosed that she was losing her eyesight. Teddi told her mother she would be too embarrassed to be there, and if she went, she would be a burden to others.

Teddi seemed to fight the notion of her increasing disabilities. She was angry about the wheelchair her parents bought. Standing up in it, at one point she shouted "No!"—the chair wasn't for her. She fell out of the chair one day, fracturing her arm. Along with her other calamities, she would also have to take a cast on her arm to Camp.

Sheri finally brought Polly in for help. Polly walked Teddi through her fears and insecurities. Some of it was hard to hear, about the boys from the year before seeing her now, the way she was, fat and disfigured. "They will laugh at me," Teddi said.

Polly let the girl talk, without interrupting and yet showing encouragement with a nod of her head or by occasionally squeezing Teddi's hand. When she felt Teddi had emptied herself of her pain and torment, Polly tackled the easier fears, the ones that could be dealt with practically.

"You liked Arts and Crafts last year," Polly said, "and you can do a lot of that this year." And sure it would be hard getting around but there were plenty of strong willing counselors at Camp who would help. "I mean, after all Teddi, that's what they're there for."

Teddi's other feelings and fears were more difficult to address or be convincing about. Both Polly and Sheri, in the days ahead, told her that many of the people at camp—campers, counselors, and staff—would be glad to see her anyway, despite all that happened to her, that her true beauty was on the inside anyway, and always.

22

The Second Camp

Both former campers, and new ones alike, were excited about being able to go to Camp Good Days and Special Times that second year. Suzie Parker felt the bus ride this time was like "leaving one world and going into another." Veteran campers could now lessen the anxiety of new campers. Laurie Allinger told a little girl nervously sitting next to her, "Don't worry—you'll be all right when you get there." Most of the counselors were back. They broke in the "greenhorns" and gave the arriving campers the same jubilant, enthusiastic reception many had received the year before.

Two people would be critical for Teddi at that Camp. One was Polly Schwensen. Polly, head counselor in Teddi's cabin, would remark that she felt as though she had gone from "a peon at the Camp the year before to Queen of the Counselors." Muggs Register would also be important to Teddi. Like Polly, she had barely come to know Teddi at Camp the year before. Muggs, arriving a few days before the campers were due to arrive, noticed Teddi off in the distance one afternoon. She was sitting in her wheelchair while adults around her talked. Even from a distance Muggs could see how much Teddi's condition had deteriorated. Muggs began to cry, by herself, for Teddi—and for the campers who would soon see and also know that Teddi was going to die.

Muggs sought out Polly. "I'll take care of Teddi," she said.

Polly wasn't sure what Muggs meant. "One-on-one you mean?"

Muggs nodded. Though most wouldn't know, this 20-year-old college student was battling Hodgkin's disease. There was a lot of spunk inside of Muggs too. "She'll need plenty of looking after," she said, matter-of-factly.

Polly nodded, and then Muggs began to walk away. Polly called out, "Thanks, okay?" Muggs smiled and continued walking.

Nurse Barbara Fredette would come for the first time to that year's Camp. Whenever she saw kids at the hospital they were usually sick, and she wanted a chance to be with them when they felt and looked better, when she could be with them more as a friend rather than a nurse.

The kids she knew were glad to see her there, too. When they got off the bus they ran up to her and hugged her, pleased to see her in blue jeans and sweatshirt and not the white clothes reminiscent of a hospital stay. Some even kidded that they were going to get back at her for all the needles she had given them, and they did, too, throughout the week; putting rubber snakes in her bed, engaging her in pillow fights, waiting for her to walk beneath the second floor windows of the main cabin to bomb her with their water balloons.

Irene Matichyn also showed up for the first time that year. It had taken some doing to get her to volunteer, and mostly that came from Skip. He had talked to her throughout the year about going, walking her through her fears and feeling of not being able to be of much help to the children anyway.

But she had come. And when the children got off the bus she was prepared to greet them with wild abandon. She had been a high school cheerleader, and known for being kind of "rah rah" politically, but she had no idea what she was in for, and what was to occur next.

She couldn't speak or move when one by one they climbed down off the bus: there were those who were bald, one who was blind, a few on crutches, many looked emaciated, one had an arm in a sling. Laurie Allinger then climbed down from the bus and for an instant Irene didn't notice that Laurie didn't have an arm. When she did see, Irene began to lose her self-control. "This is crazy," she thought to herself. "Life is crazy. How could God do this? Dear God," she cried, "how did this happen?"

Skip, watching her, came up beside her. Irene's knees were buckling and Skip helped her to the bleachers, a little distance away. All the while he talked to her. "These kids are to have fun. And we're going to let them have fun. You and I and everybody else here. Period. We're going to make them laugh."

Irene looked up and thought Skip's words were tough, but tears were falling from his eyes, too. "Trust me," he said, "after a day you won't even see them as having cancer."

Irene was shaking her head, crying even more heavily now at the sight of Skip's tears. "Oh, Skip," she said, "I don't want to do this. This is crazy. I've got enough pain in my own life—I don't need any more."

Skip held tightly onto her arm. "You get this out right here," he said. "Get this out. Don't feel sorry for them. You only have to do one thing— make sure they have a hell of a great time. That's it. And you're the kind of person who can do just that, Irene."

Irene dove into the Camp's activities with the same spirit that she showed for other endeavors. She volunteered to participate in the banana eating contest, was a major instigator for flour and cake wars, even abandoned putting make-up on each day. No self-consciousness in her corner of the world. Each night, she recalled, she went to bed utterly and totally exhausted.

Most of those who came to Camp that second year, veterans or novices, were uncertain as to how they should respond to Teddi's plainly deteriorated condition. Her "blood sisters," all in good health, came by to talk with her each day either in Teddi's cabin, at dinner, or during some of the Camp's activities. But Teddi couldn't hear very well. Laurie was too embarrassed for Teddi to shout what she was saying, and she walked away sometimes knowing that Teddi hadn't heard much, if anything, of what she had said.

Teddi required almost around-the-clock attention and by mid-week, Muggs Register was getting worn out. Teddi spent a lot of time in her cabin, away from the others, saying she was tired. Sheri thought Teddi's medication might be making her even more lethargic than usual. Changes in dosage didn't seem to help much, however. Often, they relied on counselor Jim Menz, a very strong and cooperative college student, to carry Teddi places in his arms.

Muggs went over to Polly one morning, near the flagpole, during flag-raising. "I need to talk with you," was all she said. Before Polly could say anything, Muggs began to cry.

She told Polly she was physically tired and that she was emotionally mixed-up, too. She wanted to be with Teddi all the time, to help, to cheer her up, but sometimes she just wanted to be alone, or to laugh and be with others. She knew Teddi was dying and didn't want her to die, but because of the pain Teddi was in, and how now extremely difficult daily living had become for her, Muggs sometimes felt that death might be a welcome thing.

While the others were at breakfast, Polly and Muggs walked in the woods. Polly later said that Muggs "cried and cried and cried."

The other campers would try to get Teddi involved in some of the activities. One time, when a bunch of them were going into town, they invited Teddi along. She shook her head.

"We can wheel you, Teddi," Muggs said.

"But I'm too heavy," Teddi answered.

"We'll take turns," said Polly.

Teddi still refused, and then later, Muggs, Polly, and Teddi, alone in the cabin, heard some commotion outside. Then the cabin door swung open and a crowd of boys and girls came inside singing, "We love you, Teddi—oh yes we do" over and over again. It gave Teddi all the encouragement she needed to go with them.

Skip would see Teddi at times and think she was having flash-backs of the year before. Sometimes when he was out on the dock alone, he would remember how he sang "The Rainbow Connection" with her, that spring afternoon, and the words about a voice calling her name.

What Teddi could see in memory would now have to compensate for her steadily declining vision. On the beachfront one night Sheri said, "Look at the sunset, Teddi. Isn't it beautiful?"

Teddi strained to see but told her mother it was mostly gray to her.

Seeing God's infinite wisdom in the finite life of Teddi had also become extremely difficult. One afternoon, as Sheri, along with Irene, was wheeling Teddi over a hill, the chair became stuck on a rock.

"Why does He hate me?" Teddi started to cry. "What did I ever do to Him?"

It was a warm, sunny day and around them children laughed and played. Irene moved behind the chair so Teddi wouldn't see her. She was angry with God, too.

Sheri struggled to free the chair. "God doesn't hate you, honey," she was saying. "He loves you."

"Why is He picking on me then?" Teddi wanted to know. Then she repeated new lines in her life: "Why me? Why me?"

Teddi's emotions bounced back and forth between anger and acceptance. Nurse Barb Fredette spent a brief moment with Teddi one afternoon. She sat with Teddi beneath a tall pine tree on the water's edge.

"They're having fun, aren't they, Barb?" she said.

Barb looked around at the kids, smiled, and nodded her head.

"It's sad that so many of them are sick, isn't it?" Teddi added. "But it's okay they're having fun."

Barb, a quiet person, nodded agreement without saying anything. She was content to sit with Teddi, listening to the sound of the children, and the waves lapping on the shore.

Teddi said, finally, "You know Barb, I know I'll be okay but I'm worried about my parents. If they are going to be all right."

It was the second time Teddi had said this to Barb, She was going to ask Teddi what she meant but some other children came up to her then, just to kiss Teddi, and ran away. Barb waited and Teddi seemed to go far away, too, inside, and Barb let her go.

Late in the week the entire Camp went to Lake Placid. Teddi went on the bus. They had a great time but it was a very hot day and as they were about to head back to Camp, Nurse Barb Fredette fainted. She and Teddi returned with Gary in the van.

When Barb awakened, Teddi's arm was around her. She was also holding Barb's head, looking at her and smiling. "Hi, how are you feeling?" Teddi asked.

"A lot better Teddi," Barb answered, "now that I'm next to you."

Teddi beamed. "I feel a lot better with you next to me, too, Barb." Then Teddi said, "I love you, Barb. You can tell Anne that I love her too, even though she didn't come to Camp this year. I love both you nurses. I love my daddy, too."

Gary, listening, began to smile.

Teddi yelled to him, "I love you, too, dad!"

Gary was grinning now. "I love you, too!" he called back.

Then, for the next several miles, Teddi and her father answered each other's "I love you" with another one.

The last night of Camp there was a softball game and Teddi sat in her chair, at the field's edge, watching. She told Polly that she wanted to go back to the cabin.

"Let's go for a walk instead," Polly said. "On the way back to the cabin, let's go out on the dock for awhile, okay?"

They sat there on the dock for a few moments in silence. It was twilight now, and the children in the distance were but echoes. Then squabbling, rowdy ducks broke through their own individual reflections.

"Do you want to feed the ducks, Teddi?" Polly asked.

Teddi said she'd like that, and Polly ran to the dining room for some bread. She broke it up for Teddi to throw in, which she could, with her good arm. The ducks cut through the water toward Teddi, and the bread, making the two of them laugh.

Polly didn't think Teddi had much fun that week but now, with the beauty of the night, the happy ducks, and the contented look on Teddi's face, everything seemed all right with the world. Teddi said she'd have to go to the bathroom soon and Polly nodded. Wanting to extend the happiness a little further, she went for more bread instead.

Again she broke the bread up for Teddi and Teddi threw it in, much to the delight of the ducks. Teddi, ever patient, finally couldn't hold it in anymore. "Polly, this is really fun," she said, "but I *really* do have to go to the bathroom!"

In her satisfaction, Polly had completely forgotten. Now, she raced Teddi back to the cabin, both of them laughing so hard that they cried.

Skip improved and expanded his fishing operations at Camp that year. No longer did the children have to fish from the dock; he brought his boat to take them deep water fishing. Skip held a variety of fishing contests, and on the last night of Camp would distribute awards.

A young boy named Chuckie Altamara became one of Skip's steadfast fishing companions. Chuckie fished whenever he could. He also would go on the boat when skip hunted for the small pan fish which provided so much fun for the campers.

The fishing contest held on the last day of Camp was for the biggest fish. Despite his constant attention to fishing, Chuckie didn't even catch a single one that day. At supper, he was crestfallen. But, like many kids with cancer, there is a swift emotional maturing, and considerable courage.

Chuckie, in a wheelchair like Teddi, wanted to walk from the front door of the dining hall to his table. Phil Rivaldo, who worked at Xerox Corporation and was one of the funniest of all the adults at Camp, was Chuckie's main counselor. "Go for it," he told the boy.

One by one people noticed. One by one their conversations stopped as all eyes turned toward Chuckie, slowly, unsteadily, but without help, walk to his place at one of the tables. Then the dining hall erupted. People banged forks, pounded their feet, clapped and cheered, and cried. At Camp Good Days and Special Times the small things were big, and the seemingly big things didn't matter at all.

After supper, awards were presented. One award, presented by Skip that night, was for the person who caught the biggest fish that day. As Skip talked, he could see Chuckie, cap on, with his head down. After giving out all the awards for all the contests that week, Skip said he still had one more, a special one.

"You kids go out there on the boat and catch those fish, but I'll tell you something—there was somebody who was out on the water first and who found them for you. It's hot out there and finding those fish takes a lot of time. Sometimes you even miss a lot of the activities. So this year, to my special fishing guide, I'd like to present a new rod and reel."

Chuckie slowly began to raise his head. Again, Skip walking toward him, the dining hall erupted in cheering and applause. And the two of them hugged, man and boy, for moments together that would last a lifetime.

Phil Rivaldo sat with Chuckie afterward, after everybody had stopped by to congratulate Chuckie for his award and had left the dining room. "I don't know what I can do for you, Phil," said the boy, "for all you did for me this week."

Phil pointed at the boy's sneakers. "See those?" he said.

"Yeah," Chuckie answered, bewildered.

"What you can do for me is wear them out by next year, okay?"

Chuckie promised, but it was more his heart than his body talking. After Camp Chuckie's condition worsened. Teddi would ask about him and Cheryl DeBiase thought it might be a good idea to get the two children together. "How about you two come over here for lunch," Sandy Altamura offered.

Teddi, ever the tease, had as her first line for Chuckie when she saw him, "So—what's your biggest complaint."

As Autumn slipped by that year, Teddi, who had asked how Chuckie was doing, asked less and less. Skip went to see him, and though there was snow on the ground, next to Chuckie's bed was the new rod and reel the boy would never have a chance to use. Chuckie died in November, though nobody had the heart to tell Teddi. Even when his mother came to visit Teddi, and the little girl asked how Chuckie was doing, Sandy Altamura would say that he was doing fine. That spring, the kids at the school Chuckie had gone to raised more than $10,000 as a donation to Camp Good Days and Special Times—at the time one of the largest single donations to the Camp.

On the last night of Camp, Skip DeBiase saw Irene standing alone. He took her by the arm. "Come," he said, "walk with me." And together they walked on the beach. After a few moments Skip stopped and turned to her. "Well?" he asked.

Tears once again formed in her eyes. "You were right. Make'em laugh. And I did make'em laugh, didn't I Skipper?"

Skip wanted to know how she felt.

"I can't describe it," answered Irene.

Skip said, "Now you understand."

Irene couldn't bring herself to stay to the end and say good-bye once Camp was over. "I escaped," she would later say, "in the dead of night."

That second Camp farewell was even more overwhelming than the first, and a lot of it had to do with Teddi. Her "blood sisters," one by one, gave Teddi a hug. "See you next year!" they said, loudly, so Teddi could hear them. Laurie Allinger said: "You're going to be here next year, right? Right Teddi?" She said it over and over again, with increasing intensity, almost pleading now. "I'll be here," Teddi said, finally, managing a smile.

Barb Fredette kissed Teddi good-bye. "I love you, Teddi," she whispered into Teddi's ear. "Thanks for taking care of me."

"Thanks for taking care of me, Barb," Teddi answered.

There were no boyfriends waving back to her this year, and Teddi watched, mostly silent, as the buses rolled out. Muggs was one of the last to leave. She didn't remember saying anything important or special when she said good-bye to Teddi that day. Muggs knew Teddi wouldn't be back the next year. She gave Teddi a hug and said, "I'll see you later." Once in the car, Muggs cried the distance home.

23

As Autumn Approached

Karen Lenio, Teddi's tutor, had followed developments at that second year of Camp Good Days and Special Times in the newspapers. The stories sometimes carried Teddi's picture, and so Karen could see Teddi's steady decline. Karen was to come back in the fall, even though her teaching credentials were good for grades one through six only. Nobody seemed to mind, not even officials at Teddi's school. There wouldn't be any promotion to the seventh grade.

Despite waning hope, Karen and some of the other teachers nevertheless thought it would be good for Teddi to visit the school and be a part of seventh grade for however long she could. Despite Teddi's awareness of her own appearance, the child was exuberant.

"First," she announced to her mother, "I'll go to English class."

"Whoa," said Sheri. "Now let's talk this over."

"What's there to talk over?" Teddi wanted to know.

"Do you think English class is a good idea, Teddi," asked her mother. "I mean you can't see to read and you can't hear well either."

"Then I'll sit in the front of the class," the child answered. Teddi then hemmed and hawed momentarily, adding, "I'll take a tape recorder."

"If you take that class and a lot of others, how are you going to get around? Get from class to class?"

Teddi said her friends would push her.

"Suppose they aren't going to the same class as you are?"

Miffed, Teddi said, "Well—we'll work things out then."

Teddi had a day nurse beginning early that September. Sheri wanted to know what the nurse, Laurie Freeman, was going to do if Teddi was at school all day.

"Who knows," Teddi shot back, "maybe Laurie needs some more education!"

Sheri wasn't trying to discourage Teddi, she just knew Teddi's limits in terms of care and physical endurance. Sheri was against getting Teddi's hopes up anymore. Sheri had seen the emotional devastation it had caused her daughter before. It meant, as well, that Teddi's disappointment and pain were added to Sheri's own.

It was decided, but not without some pulling of teeth, that Teddi would start with one class, art, and if that went okay, maybe other courses could be added. It was also decided that Teddi should have a tour of the school, the tour she missed that spring, prior to going. Later in the afternoon before she was to go, Teddi, Laurie, Karen, and Sheri arrived at the school.

Most of Teddi's teachers, knowing she was coming, had waited. What surprised the visitors, however, was how many of the students—also hearing Teddi was coming—had waited as well. Teddi was becoming a celebrity of sorts, maybe even a symbol for children with cancer, and her friends and kids she didn't know wanted to see her in the flesh. Karen Lenio remembers that when the tour was over that afternoon, they had quite a procession of students and teachers following them.

Even after she started school, other students would stop her in the hallway and introduce themselves. They'd offer to help with her wheelchair or with her homework. They would come into art class, knowing she would be there, just to say hello and ask how she was doing.

Teddi hadn't lost her perspective, or sense of humor, in regards to all the attention she was receiving. For instance, one little boy, also in a wheelchair, came by her and talked one afternoon. Wheelchairs can be extremely un-comfortable, and when the boy left, Teddi said to Laurie her nurse, in a loud whisper, "I wonder if his keyster gets sore, too!" Then Teddi laughed, in that infectious way she had, sending Laurie and others close by into fits of laughter as well.

But that Autumn it became increasingly difficult for Karen Lenio to find schoolwork Teddi could do. Teddi's eyesight was steadily declining, and sometimes Karen had to put one math problem on an entire page in order for Teddi to see it. Karen took to making posters for a while for information Teddi needed. Teddi kept trying. Of the number of book reports required of seventh graders, for a time Teddi was far ahead of her class. For a time.

Karen had grown close to Teddi, like Teddi's nurses at the hospital, and love and sadness are hard on the heart. To help herself endure the pain, Karen began to keep a journal. It was a way to get things out. As Autumn passed and Christmas approached, Karen Lenio made the following journal entry:

> . . . Teddi was trying as hard as ever but was extremely confused, vague, forgetful and distracted. She isn't sure what day it is, what time it is, nor whether or not she has eaten lately. She is worried about everyone, and is out of control on such things as going to the bathroom. . . . I see blue hospital baby pads under her. She gave a blood-curdling scream from the bathroom with

Laurie (the day nurse) and whimpered her way down the hall. It is heart-breaking. My dear Teddi . . . may tomorrow be better, please Lord.

That fall, Gary, Sheri, and their other children tried to make things as pleasurable as possible for Teddi. Sometimes they would make a big thing out of watching TV on Saturdays, or when there was a special program, so that Teddi had something to look forward to. They bought Walt Disney movies for her and made a fuss about making popcorn and getting ready, just like they were going out for a movie.

Other times, they would help Teddi into her favorite brown chair, put her feet on the hassock so she was comfortable, and bundle her chilly body up with blankets and pillows, sit next to her, and read. Sheri couldn't read long without her voice getting hoarse, and so the task largely fell to Gary. He would buy books or borrow them from the library that Teddi could relate to: there was the story about a blind girl confined to wheelchair; a girl who fell in love; stories about God. For the longest time, as well, Teddi wanted to keep up with her book reports, and even though she couldn't read them anymore, Gary would read them to her. Then they would do the book reports together. Together they even complained to Karen once how she only gave them a "B" for all their hard work.

A secret dread began to creep inside Sheri's heart that Autumn. She thought Teddi needed to talk to somebody who knew about religion, a priest or somebody like that, in order to find a measure of peace before she died. Sheri knew that deep inside Teddi was troubled. Sheri also feared, and this was something she came to slowly, that if Teddi died without being baptized, she might go to that place between heaven and hell Christians call "limbo." Sheri believed that Teddi might have to stay there for eternity without seeing God, and without seeing people Teddi loved. There would be no way, if this happened, for Sheri ever to find Teddi again.

Shy and watchful, there was a man who sometimes came to family court where Sheri worked whom she had come to like and respect. Warm and easy-going, Dave Ambuske was an advocate for children, heading up the Society for the Prevention of Cruelty to Children in Rochester. Ambuske was also an Anglican priest.

Father Ambuske held some strong, independent opinions about his calling that the Mervises would find out about later. As a worker-priest in France, he had come to believe that a cleric must not remain isolated or aloof from the harsh realities of the world but participate in them fully, embracing and experiencing the same pain, fear, and anguish that beset the daily lives of those who came to him for counsel and comfort. Though Sheri wouldn't know, that day when she asked for his help, the priest believed that honesty was a prerequisite in all matters of faith—even if a child was involved, even if a child was dying.

Father Ambuske's life had been nudged in the direction of Teddi's life even before he, Sheri, or Teddi knew. It began during one of his church services, when a member of the congregation said they should pray for a sick child. Over the weeks, the parishioner added more and more bits of information, like the fact that the child had a brain tumor. And then one morning, before the service started, the priest saw the woman and asked her for the name of the child. "That would mean so much more to us," he said, "to have the child's name."

"Her name is Teddi," said the woman, and from then on they prayed for a child named Teddi.

Sheri introduced herself to the priest late one Autumn afternoon. They sat beside each other on a wooden bench in the back of the empty courtroom. Sheri looked over at him only when she wanted to be sure of his reaction. This happened at the end of their conversation, when she had told him all about Teddi, and then he explained how his congregation had already begun praying for her. Sheri had asked, her voice trembling, if Dave—she called him Dave—would mind being Teddi's priest. "It would be just for a little while," Sheri said, her face red and tears squirting from her eyes.

She heard him say that of course he would do it. "Of course," he repeated. "I will be glad to come."

24

A New Friend

Father Ambuske drove to the Mervis home for the first time, thinking about what he might find. He had consulted the medical library about Teddi's particular form of cancer. He had learned about its nature, its manner of growth, and the possible side effects of treatment. From what Sheri had told him, he wasn't sure whether Teddi would want to talk to him at all. "Maybe she'll be so depressed—or angry—I won't be of much use to her," he worried. "Maybe she won't want to talk about death at all."

As he pulled into the Mervis driveway, his perspective returned to him. "Whatever happens," he told himself, "she's still just a kid. In spite of everything happening to her, she has the same attitudes and needs as any child."

Ambuske was straightforward and direct; so was Teddi. After introducing himself, he asked Teddi if she would like some time together when just the two of them were in the room. "This will be the time that's reserved for just you and me, and you can say anything you want and I won't tell anybody afterward if you don't want me to. And if we don't have anything to talk about, then it'll be our quiet time together."

Teddi said that would be fine with her except she wondered if "Sweet'ums," her pet bulldog, could also stay.

Dave laughed, telling her he liked bulldogs. "But you know what, Teddi," he told her, "I like horses best."

Teddi liked horses and Dave showed her pictures of the two he owned. "This one is named Minerva," he said, "and that's Cassie—or really—Cassiopia."

Teddi thought their names were funny.

"They're named after Greek goddesses," Dave explained. "Minerva is the goddess of wisdom, and Casseopia is the rocking chair goddess up in the sky. You can see her in the stars."

They talked about goddesses, and about horses some more, and then there was a silence. Dave asked with his eyes if it was all right to shut the door. Teddi nodded.

He thought maybe they were ready to begin. Gently as possible, he asked how she felt being sick.

The question triggered an immediate emotional reaction in Teddi. At the least, it could be the beginning of trust.

"You know," she said, "everything is always so nice for everybody. I feel sorry for myself that I'm sick and there's so much to do and I can't do it."

Dave handed her his handkerchief.

"I want to know why, Dave," she said. "Why me? Let's have some answers to that question."

His years of theological schooling, and experience as a priest, now boiled down to who and what he was as a person inside. "Well, I'll tell you something, Teddi," he said, leaning close to her and taking her hand. She lay very still on the bed, eyes looking directly into his.

"I believe something, even though I can't prove it. A lot of religion—a lot of things connected with God require our belief. It takes faith because we can talk to God all we want but we don't always get answers. And sometimes the answers we get, or think we get, are not the answers we want."

Teddi watched his eyes carefully. It was clear she wanted him to continue.

"It takes a lot of faith," he said. "Faith is what it's all about. I always believe that people like yourself get sick because there is a very special reason. And I think God picks certain people that He feels can accept that sickness and can do things with it and not just sit around and feel sorry for themselves all the time."

Teddi asked him questions about faith—what it meant, how it applied to her, what Dave meant when he talked about God's will. They talked about the fact that Teddi herself spent a lot of time thinking about other children with cancer.

She corresponded with some, she told him. And she talked to even more on the phone.

"There," Dave said, "see, you're doing just what I've said. You're thinking about others. You're accepting your sickness. You're accepting the other person's sickness but you're living as normal a life as you possibly can. I think that's the way we should live our lives, even though we know we're going to die."

Some moments passed as Dave waited to see if Teddi had more questions before he dove forward again. As he waited, he became aware of how loud the clock sounded ticking away beside Teddi's bed.

"In one sense," he continued, "you're very lucky because you know you're going to die. I don't and most people don't. I could walk out of here and drop dead. But you know you're sick and you know it's the kind of sickness that at the end—" and here he paused, just long enough for Teddi to notice, "at the end of the sickness is death. That there's no cure."

He stopped, concerned about the effect his words might have on Teddi. Teddi nodded her head. "I know," she said.

"Did you tell your mother that?" he asked.

"No," Teddi answered.

The priest wanted to know why.

"Because I don't think she could stand it," Teddi said.

Dave knew he was talking loudly but he couldn't hold back the emotion. "You're telling me you know you're going to die?"

Teddi said yes.

"But why are you telling me, Teddi?"

"Because you're supposed to know, aren't you Dave?" she answered. "You're a God-person."

Ambuske was surprised by her response. He said it sounded as though she had been giving a lot of thought to such things. She nodded that she had.

During the next several visits the priest would try to come with new jokes and stories to tell her. If he forgot, and used something he had told her before, she would stop him unhesitatingly. "C'mon now, Dave," she would tell him. "You said that before."

He would tell her how sharp she was, and then proceed to stories about the traveling he had done both in the United States and abroad. Teddi seemed to like to hear these stories, about the things he had done and the people he had met. They talked about horses a lot, too. And they talked about God and about death.

Teddi always seemed to get around to the tough theological questions just before their time together was over. She asked questions that the priest increasingly answered with use of the words "faith" and "mystery."

More time elapsed, and on one visit Teddi asked her priest how death would come for her.

Ambuske was grateful he had done his homework, and that he had inquired of his doctor friends about Teddi's ultimate physical fate. "First," he said, "there will be some difficulties. You're going to lose your hearing a little more. And you'll probably lose your sight."

He went slowly, judging with each step how much pain he might be inflicting. "Then," he said, "you're not going to be able to get up much. You're going to have to stay in bed when it gets closer and closer."

She wanted to know what came next.

"Next," he answered, reaching down inside himself for strength, "next— it will probably be a coma, Teddi. Most likely you'll stay in a coma, and go to sleep that way, and die. That's not going to be painful for you. All the pain you've had will be behind you then."

On his next visit, Teddi's theological question for the day was about heaven. She wanted Dave to tell her what it would be like. Would, for example, God have a beard like the pictures she had seen?

"That will be a surprise," he said, smiling, and having come to know how much Teddi liked surprises.

She now had a surprise for him. "I'll find out the answer to that question, and some of the others, before you will, won't I Dave?"

He nodded his head. "You probably will, Teddi."

Dave broke the silence that followed. He asked Teddi if she would deliver some messages to God for him. He told her things about his mother. Things about God he wondered about. And she told him she would take what he said and bring it with her, bring all of it with her when she saw God.

Autumn came early that year, it had come all too quickly for those who knew how it felt to be with long winters. On one such cold afternoon, as Dave was about to leave, Teddi asked him the specifics of her death. "What will happen when I die, Dave, here I mean?"

Ambuske explained that there would be a funeral and that they would bring Teddi's body into the church. Then they would pray over her body. He also said it was customary for the priest to talk about the person who died. "It's called a eulogy, Teddi," he explained. "And after the eulogy there will be more prayers and some music maybe."

"And there will be lots of people there," he said, trying to lighten the burden of what he was saying. "Lots of people will come because they love you and your family."

"In the church, Dave?" she wanted to know. "They'll come to the church?"

"That's right, Teddi, people will come to the church, and I will probably say a few words about you."

Teddi scrunched her shoulders and clasped her hands. "And?" she said, waiting.

"And?" Dave repeated, uncertain.

"And what will you say about me?"

"Oh, I'll tell them what a wonderful person you are," he said. "How you did things for others. How you dealt with your suffering without complaining. I'll tell them about your love of animals and your love of people. I'll tell them about some of the things we talked about—I mean—if that's okay with you."

She told him it would be all right to talk about those things then.

Teddi broke the silence this time.

"Do you remember telling me about how you saw the Sistine Chapel, Dave," she began. "And how there's the picture of God and his finger is touching Adam's?"

Ambuske nodded.

"I'd like to feel that I was like that. That I touched a lot of people."

"Oh, you have," Ambuske joined in. "You have, Teddi. With the Camp, you've touched a lot of people. Not only the kids, but all the people who know about it and helped it along."

The sudden rush of enthusiasm was once again followed by silence. It had grown dark in the room, but neither of them seemed to notice or care.

"Will you be sad, Dave," came the sound of Teddi's voice. "Will you be sad when you talk about me?"

In all the time he had been with her, the priest never cried. He turned toward the window, then back again to her. "Of course I will be sad, Teddi," his voice faltering and just above a whisper. "I love you and will miss you very much. So will everybody who knows you."

"I don't want you to be sad, though, Dave," Teddi said. "If you cry then so will my mom and dad. I don't want them to cry. It's not like good-bye. I don't like good-byes. I'm leaving one side and going to another, aren't I? It's more like hello than good-bye then, isn't it?"

The priest, comforted, said, "You're right. Of course you're right, Teddi."

She told him, toward the end of their time together, that she wanted her funeral to be a happy time.

On every other occasion when he left, Dave would try to leave Teddi with a smile. He would call her "Lizzie"—and pick out other names. That day, as he left—and all the days he had with her hence—he said, "I'll see you later, pretty lady."

"Pretty lady?" Teddi said.

"Yes," he answered. " 'Pretty lady.' Because that's what you are and that's what you'll always be to me."

Teddi wanted to understand better and more. "But I've lost my hair," she said. "And you know I've got a scar."

"That's not you," said the priest. "I see what you are on the inside, the *real* you, the you that will live on forever and ever . . . "

25

Hope Rethought

The next visit Dave Ambuske paid to Teddi Mervis began with a request. Teddi asked the priest if she could be baptized.

Ambuske was pleased and smiled. Still, he wondered if Teddi thought baptism might cure her, or transform her physical appearance. "You'll be a child of God," he told her gently, "but you might not notice any physical change."

She nodded. "I know, Dave," she said, "but I would like it anyway."

That evening, Teddi talked over the possible baptism with her parents. They were happy for her and approved. Yet the doubt began to form inside them, as it had with the priest, that Teddi wanted the baptism because she believed it might somehow alter her fate. Afterward, Teddi asked her mother is if she would dial the DeBiase number. Cheryl answered.

"I'm going to be baptized, Cheryl," Teddi exclaimed proudly. "And I would like you to be my godmother."

Cheryl was grateful the conversation was taking place on the telephone, for she began to cry. "I'd be happy to," she said, covering up the receiver.

"Can you put Skipper on?" Teddi wanted to know.

A phone call, given Teddi's condition, was cause for concern in the DeBiase home. Skip had come into the room right after Cheryl started talking. He feared for the worst. Now he took the phone Cheryl was handing him. "Teddi's got something to ask you," she said, and left the room.

Teddi told Skip about wanting to be baptized, and tears formed in his eyes. For some reason, thoughts of the Last Rites, a Catholic sacrament for dying persons, had come to mind. She asked him to be her godfather and he said yes, he'd be honored to.

"I'll be almost Italian now, won't I?" she joked.

But Skip was serious. "You'll be what's called my 'comare'—and that's being as close as you can get without being blood."

Before bed, Sheri told Teddi it was customary, with baptism, for the recipient to select a new name. Teddi said she wanted the name "Angelina"— which in Italian meant "little angel." Many of the Mervis friends were Italian and used to kid her that she looked more like an Italian than any other nationality. Now, when they heard the name she picked, they would tell her she belonged more to them than to anybody.

The day of the baptism approached and Teddi became increasingly excited. She had a hard time even taking her afternoon naps. She and her mother made a cake for that day and had to try a few times in order to get "Elizabeth Angelina Mervis" on its top. Teddi also picked out a new white dress for the occasion. With her eyesight failing, she asked her mother now and again if she herself could feel the material.

On the day of the baptism Sheri put pink ribbons in her daughter's wig. As she folded and tied them she asked Teddi a question that had been bothering her ever since the child said she wanted to be baptized. Did she, her mother wanted to know, expect the baptism to change her in any way?

Teddi, whose voice was low now and who spoke haltingly said she didn't expect anything to change about her body or her tumor. "I'm just so excited about doing this," she said. "This is more exciting than Christmas."

Sheri smiled. She was convinced now that it wasn't just having a party or getting gifts that had motivated Teddi. Sheri felt her Autumn wish of asking Father Ambuske for help had been realized. Teddi was accepting God, she thought, and God would also be welcoming her.

As family and close friends arrived that day they remarked to Teddi, and to one another, then and later, how beautiful she looked and how she seemed to glow. Photographs of the event confirm the way her face seemed to beam, as if something peaceful and good was happening inside.

"C'mon everybody," Teddi called out in the noisy room, "let's get this show on the road!"

Father Ambuske explained that Teddi was going to have to repeat after him. Then he turned to the crowd and gave a detailed description of what was to follow, and what it signified. Turning back to Teddi, he asked if she was ready.

Into the mood of the occasion, Teddi wanted to know if she was to repeat everything he told people about the ceremony! Everybody laughed, including the priest, who felt at that moment their deep and abiding friendship.

Those gathered watched quietly and intently. Some, like Irene Matichyn, moved to the back of the crowd because she could feel herself starting to cry, and she didn't want to spoil the occasion. At the end of the brief ceremony, they all clapped their approval. Gary uncorked a bottle of champagne and each person present took turns kissing Teddi and telling her how lovely she looked and how beautiful the ceremony was. Each also had come with a gift.

Irene, toward the end of the line, handed Teddi several pounds of cashew nuts. "My dad will eat them, too!" Teddi said, trying, it seemed, to make Irene laugh. No, Irene answered, Gary wasn't to have any.

Skip, Teddi's godfather, was the last to present his gift. Though the others were milling about now, talking, the room swiftly grew silent as Skip placed a gold necklace in her hand and explained what the heart, anchor, and dove signified.

"It's from Italy," he told her, and she nodded, happily. He told her that the heart is for love and it was because she was the kindest person he knew. "The anchor is for faith," he said, "and your baptism is proof of that."

He held the dove now and realized he should have thought about what he was saying before, before he started, before Teddi and all those present were waiting and listening.

"The dove is for hope, comare," he said, finally, putting hope in a different place altogether now. "And you've brought more hope to kids than anybody I know."

After the baptism, Father Ambuske continued to come by for his weekly visits with Teddi. When Teddi was feeling well they would chat and discuss their heavy theological questions. When Teddi was sick, he sometimes sat there holding her hand, praying for her and the children like her.

Teddi was no longer able to walk, or even stand by herself. Her weight increased even more. And the optometrist told Sheri not to be optimistic about Teddi's eyesight remaining stable or reversing itself. After one of his visits, Teddi's pediatrician, Dr. Nazarian, wrote in his report that Teddi "gets depressed." He also commented that she has "some good days" however.

Father Ambuske was concerned about Teddi's impending blindness and wanted to deal with it realistically and with some positive good coming out of it. After telling her that her eyesight would continue to fail, he asked if she would close her eyes. Then the priest described the sky outside her window, what the trees looked like, and what the wind was doing to them. Teddi then opened her eyes to compare what she had imagined with what she was able to see.

"You have an advantage over many blind people," Dave told her. "You know what things looked like, and what color is, and you can remember them."

That day, and on the visits that followed, the priest trained the child in identifying colors, in being able to hold onto pictures of the world outside, and of him, her siblings, and her mother and father.

On a cold crisp Autumn day Ambuske entered her room and greeted her. She was somewhat reticent. The afternoon sun had set and Ambuske reached for her bedside lamp to turn it on. Something made him stop. He pulled back his hand and then pulled up his chair. He took her hand.

"You can't see me, can you Teddi?" he said.

She shook her head.

"Can you see anymore?"

"No, no I can't Dave," she whispered.

And so Father Ambuske, from that day forward, described Teddi's world in the colors she had learned and the images imprinted upon her mind. He would tell her what the sky looked like, and the trees, and what the wind was doing with the snow.

A favorite thing Teddi would ask the priest, at the outset of each visit after that, was which color suit he was wearing.

"It's the brown one," he might say.

And Teddi might pop back with, "Oh, no, Dave, you wore that suit last time. Not too much now."

And the priest would be cheered.

Sometimes, some of Teddi's old sad questions returned. "Why me?" she'd sometimes ask, and Father Ambuske would patiently start at the beginning, with the answers from the first day they met, even though they were nearing the end of their time together.

Because of her blindness, the strong medication, and her own personal disorientation and fears, Teddi's care became increasingly difficult and fatiguing. Teddi wouldn't know what time it was anymore and would call out in the middle of the night sometimes for help. When Sheri or one of the others got to her room, she sometimes forgot what she had called them for. Often, she just wanted to be turned, her back or her arm or leg ached from being in the same place too long.

Tod would come by each morning before school and call into the room. "Hey, Teddi, what are you doing in bed again?"

"Hi, dad," Teddi would sometimes answer.

Those times, teasing Tod would sit on the bed next to her without saying anything. Teddi, who could tell by the weight it wasn't her father, would reach out and try to poke Tod. "Oh, Tod," she'd tell her brother, "you're such a joker! You're always trying to trick me!"

Toward the end of November, late one afternoon, Teddi said to her mother, sitting by the bed, that a little boy had come into the room and wanted to play.

"Where is he?" Sheri wanted to know.

"Over there," Teddi told her, pointing to the corner of the room farthest from the door.

"What's he wearing," her mother asked, and Teddi told her the boy had a shirt on.

"Oh, okay," said Sheri, "if he wants to play, he can play."

The next day, at around the same time, Teddi said the boy was back again but this time some other boys were picking on him. "Mommy," yelled Teddi, "Quick! Help him!"

Sheri scolded the boys. "You bad kids get out of here and leave that little boy alone."

Teddi thanked her mother. "They were going to hurt him," she said.

Sheri told her daughter, "We're not going to let anybody get hurt around here." And then she asked Teddi if she knew the boy's name. Teddi said she didn't know but would ask him the next day when he came.

The next day Teddi said that the boy had come and she asked him his name but had forgotten. "Well, you think about it," said Sheri, "and let me know when you remember." She added, "Why don't you invite him for spaghetti the next time he comes by. Everybody loves spaghetti."

It was two days more before Teddi said the boy had returned. She looked sad or depressed, her mother couldn't tell which. "What's the matter, Teddi?" she asked.

Teddi was slow in answering. "He's waving for me to come with him," she said.

Sheri asked her daughter if he was a nice boy.

"Oh, yes," Teddi smiled. "He's very nice. He has a very kind face."

Sheri asked if he had told her his name yet.

"Yeah, he did," said Teddi, but she couldn't remember again.

Teddi couldn't see the tears running down her mother's cheeks. She leaned close to Teddi's face. "Teddi," she said, "Is his name Jesus?"

Teddi was excited, nodding her head up and down. "That's it, Mommy! That's his name! How did you know?"

"I was just guessing, honey," Sheri whispered.

There was a long pause, Teddi appearing as though she was already with the boy. Her mother interrupted. "Teddi," she said, and waited.

After a few moments Teddi asked what she wanted.

"Teddi," her mother said, "if you want to go with him, it's all right."

PART III

Of Death and a Dream

26

"They've Come for Teddi"

Several days later, Teddi asked her mother to box up and put away all her teddy bears. Sheri wanted to know why.

"I'm too old now," Teddi said.

Her mother tried to convince her to keep them out. "You've got so many and you've loved them so much," she said.

"I know, Mommy," Teddi said, "but I'm too old now."

Sheri wanted to know if she could put shelves on the wall and put all the bears there.

"They'll be in Kim's way," Teddi told her mother.

Round and around they went, Teddi finally giving up when her mother said she would try to find some boxes and begin putting them away.

It was December now and Teddi's condition was steadily worsening. Sheri called the hospital and had them deliver a bed, which was put in the living room. Sheri also talked with Teddi's pediatrician, Dr. Nazarian. She told him that Teddi was undergoing personality changes—that she was crying and complaining more—and also calling for her for no apparent reason. Sheri told Nazarian that Teddi slept a great deal now and seldom left her bed.

Nazarian came by to examine Teddi a few days before Christmas. According to his notes of the visit, he thought Teddi was "having a good day" that day. He also wrote:

> . . . She cannot see, but she hears and understands fairly well. She answered my questions with one or a few word answers. She told one joke in somewhat halting, sometimes indistinct words. She ate pancakes and sausage, slowly, when fed by the nurse Laurie Freeman. She seems to drift into a quiet almost sleep-like state quite often, but will then suddenly make a clear request. After going to bed, she cried out frequently for her mother. She screamed when we tried to take her blood pressure and said it hurt a great deal.

Friends came by to see her during the holidays, and then the time for the second annual Camp Christmas party arrived. Teddi didn't want to go at first. She was practically immobile at that point and could barely stay awake. Her back and bottom hurt considerably even if she was in her wheelchair for a short while.

Her body hurt so much that soon after the Camp Christmas Party started Teddi had to lie on her sleeping bag in a corner of the room. Muggs Register lay down beside her and stayed there until the party was over.

During the party, campers came over to tell Teddi hello in her ear. Counselors came by to wish her a Merry Christmas. Teddi's "blood sisters" told her gossip and pretended, they said later, that she was not any different from before, during that first year, when they were all well and together. Some people, like nurse Barb Fredette, started to tell her something but were too overcome with grief to continue—hurriedly moving away.

One of the most troubling developments, after the party was over, was that Teddi never truly believed she was brought home afterward. She would plead with her mother to take her home, even though she was in the hospital bed and in the family living room.

"When are we going home? Please take me home. If I'm really a good girl will you promise to take me home, Mommy?" she'd plead over and over again.

Sheri would sometimes become strident. "But you are home, Teddi. Please believe me." And she would make Teddi feel her bed, the bears, the faces of friends and family.

After several days of insisting she wasn't home, Sheri got her dressed and took her in the van. They drove around before returning home. "There," said Teddi's mother, "we're home now." And she shut off the engine. "Feel the first step to the house, Teddi?" she said, helping her inside. And once inside Tod was waiting with an armful of her favorite bears. "See Teddi," he said, putting the bears in her hands and next to her face, "here's your bears. Now you've got to be sure you're home now."

No matter what they tried, Teddi believed she had left home for good. One last time, on Christmas Eve, as the family was putting up the tree, Teddi asked if she might be home by Christmas.

The day after Christmas the Mervises inquired about Hospice Care. This kind of care provides the opportunity for terminally ill patients to die at home, around loved ones and in an environment familiar to them.

Teddi was sleeping even more than usual at this point. And when Dr. Nazarian visited again in mid-January, he believed, again according to his notes, that Teddi was "becoming more somnolent (sleepy) and withdrawn."

She did have good days, however infrequently they came now. And people would come by then, getting in as much conversation as they could, for everyone knew that the time for words was growing thin. On one of Teddi's "good days," Karen Lenio came by. Her journal entry for January 15th read:

. . . She was awake today. Hooray! Not comfortable, not chatty, but AWAKE. She knew I was there, she knows I love her, she repeated "I love you, too." That's all I hoped for in a way of conversation. I could rub my lips over her cheek and touch the fuzzy top of her head. . . . And I could smell the powdery sweet smell. Like a baby. A visit for all the senses.

It was January 18th and both Sheri and Gary, coming home each day for lunch now, found Teddi's seizures frequent and intense. They called Dr. Nazarian who recommended increasing her medication. That didn't work and so Nazarian told the Mervises to take Teddi to the hospital by ambulance. Sheri rode inside the ambulance with Teddi; Gary followed from behind, being driven by home care nursing supervisor Angie Mastrodonato.

Betty Scobell was standing next to the sink that afternoon and saw the red lights reflecting in her window. Her husband then came into the room. She saw tears in his eyes.

"What's the matter?" she asked.

He shook his head. "They've come for Teddi. It's an ambulance."

Betty turned to look at the clock. It was 5:00 P.M. She was sorry it was suppertime and there would be a lot of people coming home. They would stare. "The Mervises don't need that," she said to herself.

Tod was at wrestling practice that afternoon when he saw a policeman enter the room. The coach pointed in his direction and the cop started walking toward him. "Oh, God," thought Tod, "I'm really in trouble now. What did I do?"

The policeman was a friend of Gary's who came to tell Tod what was happening and to take him to the hospital. Tod said afterward that hearing the news about his sister was worse than any trouble he could've gotten into.

When Teddi arrived at the hospital she was immediately given an I.V. of valium to help control her seizure activity and what the doctor's report described as "other movements of agitation." She had a fever. She was also put on a respirator. The doctor would also record that "the parents at this point seem near the breaking point." He closed his descriptions and recommendations for treatment that day with the phrase: "end stage tumor."

Nurses Anne, Barb, and Sally each came by to see Teddi when they reported to work. All were deeply saddened by Teddi's bloated frame and the stretch marks over her body. Teddi also didn't know who they were anymore.

Teddi slipped into what was referred to as a "light" coma, only occasionally crying out "Mama"—"Dad," that evening and early morning. Her seizure activity continued despite dosages of phenobarbitol. The side rails on her bed were left up now, and they were padded.

There was little left for doctors, nurses, and science to do. It was talked about by medical personnel and the Mervises and made clear that the purpose of this admission was to control possible infection and to make Teddi's stay as comfortable as possible. The hope now was that Teddi would be able to return home to die.

But her condition worsened even that day. She had difficulty in swallowing her own saliva. She was incontinent and diapers were used. When her fever shot up, which it often did, she was wrapped in a cooling blanket. Her left hand looked deformed now.

After Father Ambuske left, giving Teddi "Last Rites," Sheri was alone with her in the room. She put her face up close to her daughter's, whispering, "I love you, Teddi."

Then, in her last lucid moments on earth, Teddi whispered, "I love you" back.

27

Waiting

Teddi, for a while, responded to words called into her ear with a grunt. Sally Masten, the small, gutsy nurse who had lost her fiance to cancer and still continued working with cancer patients, recalled how she was nevertheless devastated one day when she went into the room to find Sheri, next to Teddi, saying over and over again, "Are you all right, honey? Do you hurt?"

Gary stayed in Teddi's hospital room the full twenty-four hours each day for the first week. He became so exhausted that Sheri, his friends, and the medical staff insisted he go home for some much needed rest. Yet even there, his thoughts were of Teddi. Watching NBC's "News Magazine," on at the time, he learned about a foundation in Phoenix, Arizona, called "Make a Wish." It was a special fund for terminally ill children so that they could have their last wish come true. He wondered about maybe setting up something like that in Rochester, and western New York, for children who were dying.

Kim and Tod would have a difficult time. Kim never talked about it much, but Tod remembered talking to Teddi about how he was doing in wrestling, and what Teddi's friends were up to at school. One night, when Teddi was worse than usual, Sheri told nurse Barb Fredette she would like to stay late. Barb volunteered to take Tod home for her. As they left the hospital together, Tod put his hand on Barb's shoulder. She turned and could see he had tears in his eyes and that he was choked up. She felt he probably didn't want her to see him that way.

"Is Teddi going to die tonight?" he asked.

Barb didn't expect the question. She told him she couldn't answer that.

On the way home, Tod talked virtually non-stop, mostly about small matters. Barb glanced over at him from time to time, and when headlights washed across his face, she could see how anxious he looked. She thought he was probably talking so much, and so fast, to prevent himself from crying.

Later, Tod would say that through Teddi's long ordeal he still thought "the Lord would come through—change things and save my sister's life."

It is generally believed that hearing is the last sense to leave when someone is in a comatose stage. And so those who loved her stayed and talked to her, even though she could no longer respond, even with a groan.

Father Ambuske continued to come by for his weekly visit, at the same time he normally had come. He told her what the sky looked like, how the trees looked like lace, and that he was wearing his blue—not his brown—suit. Bob Mervis sat alone holding Teddi's hand. Not one to talk much, he looked at Teddi and remembered thinking to himself that her life was slipping away from her now.

Barb Fredette watched the Mervises leave one night, crying, and wondered if that night was going to be Teddi's last. Teddi had been moaning a great deal and also seemed to be in a great deal of discomfort. That night, Barb gave her the maximum pain medicine recommended. She stayed late in the room, holding Teddi's hand, thinking that the Mervises would want her to be there if Teddi died.

Barb thought about God and was angry for a time. The death of children seemed such a cruel fate to this gentle, quiet nurse. But Barb Fredette knew that what kept her going, what made her stay with Teddi even now, was that she had known love. She was loved for what she was doing—and did. That past summer, when the sun was hot and the air thick, Teddi Mervis told her so over and over again in the back of a van.

To Skip DeBiase, those weeks when Teddi was in a coma were the worst of her entire sickness. "There was a point," he said, "where nothing but despair existed." Sometimes, when he became upset or overly angry, he knew it wasn't because of one thing or another, or any one person, but because he was frustrated. There was nothing anybody could do. "We're taking out our aggressions on each other," he said to his wife once, "because you can't hit God. My arms are too short to box with God."

Polly would come to Teddi's room and sit and hold her hand, despite the fact that some of the doctors said Teddi was a "vegetable" now. Polly would become angry with the doctors when they wouldn't even come into the room to check on her. They said it didn't matter any more now.

But one by one the people who loved Teddi continued to come and sit next to her. With people in the room or alone, they talked to Teddi for a while, hoping she could still hear them, hoping it pleased and comforted her to know she wasn't alone.

Gary tried to keep his own spirits up. He told Polly during this period that while he thought Teddi was doing poorly, he didn't think she was "at death's door." Sheri told Polly of her conversation with Teddi about the little boy named Jesus coming and Polly indeed agreed that Teddi was probably asking her mother's permission to die. Sheri also said that she thought this was the last part of the illness now and hoped Teddi's death would be peaceful.

Father Ambuske's congregation continued praying for Teddi, as January gave way to February. Week by week the priest would tell his parishoners how the child was doing. Sometimes, afterward, they would ask him if it was a good sign that she was still hanging on. "No," he said, "hope of her surviving is lost." And then he began to add, with an equal balance of pride and sadness, "But it shows you the strength of this child. She's very, very strong-willed."

Teddi's breathing became more labored. Suctioning was now necessary to clear her throat of a white mucous that began to form. There was less and less bodily movement. Dr. Nelson's examination of her now showed she had no reflexes. This, he thought, reflected the tumor's almost complete involvement. "Terminal stage," he wrote in Teddi's record that day, "high liability for aspiration."

On February 3rd, just after midnight, Gary came running from Teddi's room. "Barb," he yelled, "something's wrong with Teddi!" Nurse Fredette grabbed another nurse and a doctor. "This is it," she thought to herself, but disciplined her emotions. Nurse Fredette put the bag used to stimulate breathing over Teddi's mouth. She pumped it a few times and Teddi's breathing, and life, was restored. This was the third time Teddi had to be revived manually.

Laurie Allinger learned that Teddi had slipped into a coma. She called Suzie Parker in Camden, New York, and together they cried on the phone. Afterward, Laurie went to the hospital to see Teddi. She saw Sheri come out of the room crying. Sheri passed by the girl without noticing her, and Laurie couldn't bring herself to go into the room. She left without seeing her "blood sister" alive again.

Muggs Register remembered Gary asking her to stay in Teddi's room toward the end while he made a phone call. Gary didn't want Teddi to die alone, she thought. Father Ambuske told the medical staff on Teddi's floor to please call him if death was near but his message got buried in a pile of notes and messages and was lost.

No matter how much they loved and cared about Teddi, still, in each person who came and waited, there was the fear that Teddi would die when they were in the room. Anne Cameron didn't know if she could bear up and asked Polly to pray it wouldn't happen on her shift. Skip DeBiase felt that each of them, with each visit, was emotionally playing a kind of "Russian roulette."

Afterward, they would talk about being in the room alone with Teddi and looking up, anxiously, when she gasped for air. They would stare steadily and long to see some trace of movement in the white sheet draped over Teddi's body. Who would be the one, they wondered, that would be in the room when Death, like a cool breeze, would come—rustling papers, making the curtains tremble, taking Teddi's life away? Who would be the one to see this child breathe for one last time?

One afternoon, as Sheri and Anne talked, Sheri inquired about what happened to the body after somebody died.

"We clean them first," Anne answered.

"Do they have clothes on?" Sheri wanted to know, and Anne didn't have the heart to tell her that the body normally went downstairs to the hospital morgue in a plastic bag.

Sheri kept pausing, as if trying to catch her breath. And then she asked if Teddi could go downstairs to the morgue with a nightgown on.

Anne promised that she would.

28

A Child Dies

It was unusual for a child in a coma to moan but Teddi did so periodically, and it troubled people. Did she moan because she was in pain? Because she was trying to shake herself awake? Did she want something? Want to *say* something? Nurse Sally Masten, disturbed about the moaning, asked a resident physician what he thought was going on. He shook his head. "Nobody knows," he said.

One night, after moaning for several days, Teddi stopped moaning with the same suddenness in which she had started. Barb Fredette was on duty and decided to call Gary and Sheri at home to tell them, and to say that Teddi seemed to be resting peacefully now. The Mervises told her they were grateful for the news.

Sally Masten had assumed a larger role in Teddi's care. With Teddi, care at this point involved turning and changing her periodically, and continued moistening of her lips with vaseline so they wouldn't dry up and crack and bleed. Sally also made sure the curtains were open, despite the fact that Teddi couldn't see and might not even be aware. Sally hoped Teddi could feel the sun's warmth and maybe even tell that night had turned to day.

The precariousness of Teddi's life began to unlock the anger and resentment stored away in her parents. One time, for example, the Mervises had returned to Teddi's room after going out for supper only to find Teddi had wet her diapers, and that her bed was soaked. Nurse Sally Masten had left the room moments before the Mervises arrived and everything had been all right. Now the Mervises called Nurse Masten into the room, chewing her out for what they perceived as lack of attentiveness to Teddi.

Sally didn't say anything. She listened, going about her work changing Teddi's diapers and bed. A few moments passed and Gary, uneasy at what had just transpired, tried to joke with Sally. "Gee, Sal," he said, smiling, "and here we thought you were a good nurse."

Sally would have none of it. "Gary," she said, trying to remain calm, "don't joke with me. I'm very upset." She then told them that when she finished she would like to speak with them in the conference room down the hall.

Moments later, shutting the door behind her, Sally was direct with the Mervises. "I think we've got to adjust this right now," she began. "I love both of you and I love Teddi. And if this isn't adjusted right now it will cause bad feelings on both our parts. I know you're ticked at me, and I am also ticked."

Gary, still trying to smooth things over, said they weren't ticked.

Sally stuck to her concerns. "You *were* ticked, Gary," she said. "And I want you to know I give myself one-hundred percent to Teddi. If you don't think that's good enough for you then by all means look into getting another caretaker."

Gary told her that he and Sheri were both there to make certain their daughter got one-hundred percent care and if they ever thought anybody taking care of Teddi was giving less than that then they certainly would look into a replacement. But he also told Sally that he and his family loved her, and that they thought she was a very good nurse. He said they were "just very upset when we came back and found her like that."

Sally said she understood. But she told them they also had to understand that she "knew exactly where they were coming from." And then she told them about her own losses to cancer. Her father had died of cancer. Then, less than five months later, her fiance died of Hodgkin's disease. "I know how anxious you are," she said, her own painful memories rushing to the surface now, "and I know how you want to do everything you can. I understand your frustration but you must trust other people—and me—too."

Sally's courage and honesty were qualities the Mervises admired. They told her they would try. And after that, after the confrontation, they seemed to move even closer in their understanding and affection for each other. At times this came out in the form of humor.

One particular pattern involved the taking of Teddi's temperature. Sally would put a thermometer under Teddi's arm, chat a few minutes, and then go take care of a sick child. Returning to the room, whether she remembered leaving the thermometer tucked in Teddi's arm or not, she would try to remove it without being noticed. At that point, one or both the Mervises would clear their throat and ask how Teddi's temperature was doing.

The closeness of the nurse to the Mervises was brought out in other ways as well. One time, for example, Sally came into the room only to find Sheri, standing over Teddi, crying. Without saying a word, Sally moved next to where Sheri was standing, put her arm around the woman, and also began crying, too.

Dr. Nazarian, Teddi's pediatrician, came by nearly every day now. An energetic, sensitive man, he had grown fond of the Mervis family, and especially Teddi. He felt a responsibility to provide Teddi with optimal care within the means of the hospital staff. As the ordeal of Teddi's coma wore on, however, conflicting pressures began to arise and sometimes tempers even flared.

The Mervis family—and especially Gary—were very anxious about the details of Teddi's care. Worried that the medical staff was giving up on Teddi, seeing her situation as hopeless, he had asked to see copies of Teddi's medical records.

This irritated the hospital staff, who felt they weren't being trusted. Moreover, with Teddi's life so tenuous, Gary was insisting on clarity regarding resuscitation efforts. He continued to worry that if her breathing stopped, medical personnel on duty might let her die without trying anything. They explained all this to Dr. Nazarian now, seeming to bare their soul in these last final days. Gary didn't mention, though Dr. Nazarian knew anyway, that Gary would be searching for a cure or some discovery or some way to prolong Teddi's life even if it were for a little while longer.

Having experienced such situations before, Dr. Nazarian let two criteria guide him. First, he would weigh whether a proposed treatment or course of action would in fact help Teddi, or if it would cause her discomfort and be an inappropriate intrusion on her personhood. The second thing he weighed was whether plans or promises of future actions would hasten or retard her decline, even though her life at this point was measured in days and even hours.

Nazarian also believed in honesty in his approach. And to the Mervises, he wanted affirmation that they understood this was the final stage of Teddi's ordeal, and that she would in all likelihood not regain consciousness. He also told them that in his opinion, given Teddi's medical needs at that point, she would probably have to stay in the hospital rather than be able to return home.

Sheri wanted to know what was happening to Teddi on the inside and Nazarian said: "As far as we can tell Teddi's in a dream-state. Perhaps she is even seeing and hearing images and sounds in her mind with a clarity denied her by her failing senses when she was last conscious."

Gary said he wanted the medical staff to make an "honest effort" to revive Teddi if she did stop breathing. He told the doctor that Teddi was trying so hard he believed she ought to be helped. He didn't want a respirator used to revive her, or a "full code," just a modest attempt. If her heart stopped, Gary wanted them to try CPR (Coronary Pulmonary Resuscitation) or maybe some drug to try and stimulate it. Teddi should also be encouraged to breathe manually, Gary said, through the standard rubber bag used for such purposes. The doctor supported Gary in the proposed course of action and assured him that Gary's recommendations would be written into the hospital record so there would be no mistakes and no room for misinterpretation.

At that point, Nazarian remembered Sheri appeared agitated and voiced her concern that she be notified of any change in Teddi's condition. Nazarian assured her that her concern would be relayed by him to the medical staff.

As the meeting drew to a close, the conversation became more personal. The doctor listened, he remembered, as both Gary and Sheri expressed their hope that Teddi would continue to live, while at the same time acknowledging what a terrible emotional and physical toll it was taking on Teddi herself, and also on those who watched and waited.

Before he left, Nazarian told the couple he would put their concerns and recommendations in writing for the medical staff and forward a copy to them. He also asked them for patience in dealing with the health care professionals involved in Teddi's care. The focus of their study and training, he told them, was to keep people alive. With death waiting, they lacked purpose and often became overwhelmed by frustration themselves.

Nurse Sally Masten saw Gary coming out of the room after the meeting. He pulled her aside. She was surprised that she hadn't seen earlier how worn Gary had become. His voice was hoarse, like somebody who was going to cry or had just stopped. "I want to do everything I can for my daughter," he told her. "I want to make sure that everything is supplied that is support for her in case she isn't going to die."

Sally nodded. "I understand your hope," was all she could say before moving away.

One of the things Dr. Nazarian concluded in his notes of their meeting was that he found the Mervises the kind of people who were taking negative feelings and situations and trying to make something positive out of them. This was born out in a press conference called by Gary Mervis for the morning of January 29th.

The Teddi Mervis story and the inspiration of Camp Good Days and Special Times was one of western New York's most popular stories, and so the press conference was covered by the three major local television stations, by radio reporters, and received special attention in Rochester's two large daily newspapers. Many of the people involved in Teddi's care, and other children on the pediatric floor at the hospital, were watching the taped press conference that day as well.

Gary announced the establishment of the "Teddi Project" that day. He had met with the board of directors of Camp Good Days and Special Times and they had approved of a special fund to give terminally ill children a last final wish. The Board, upon the recommendation of one of its members, unanimously voted in favor of naming this special fund after Teddi Mervis.

Gary Mervis spoke without notes, talking with only a hint of emotion. He explained that "the family of a terminally ill child is dealing both with emotional frustration and economic pressures. They really didn't need the additional frustration of knowing it is beyond their wherewithal to do something special that their child might want at the end." Gary wanted these people to know there was a fund ready to help in such circumstances. This was the least the living could do, Gary said, for those whose lives were so painful and brief. And he concluded with the words that the Teddi Project would be a "living memorial to my daughter."

Teddi developed phlebitis in her left ankle because of the persistence of the I.V. tube there. After several attempts, the I.V. was moved to her wrist. Of even greater seriousness, on a few occasions she stopped breathing and had to be revived. She seemed to slip into an even deeper coma now. Her breathing became increasingly irregular, with long gasps between breaths. The moaning returned.

Dr. Nelson explained the results of another CT scan which was done. "The tumor is now massive," he told them. "It occupies about three-fourths of Teddi's right cerebral hemisphere." A few days later Gary suggested to Dr. Nelson that they try an "external ventricular drainage" or shunt. Gary thought the procedure might relieve some of the pressure on Teddi's brain. Teddi had grimaced a few times, and at one point even flashed her eyelids. Gary thought that, and the moaning, were perhaps cues she wanted him to take.

Nelson listened to Gary's recommendation with care. Before offering his opinion, he talked to Gary about the risks and complications involved, and some other options—including doing nothing. He did finally say, however, that he agreed with Gary that a shunt might relieve some of the pressure on her brain. He also said he'd be willing to perform the procedure if that was Gary's desire.

Next morning, after dressing, Gary looked through his dresser drawer for a handkerchief. He took one with him to the hospital every day now. He found the one Teddi had given him for Christmas and hoped it would bring him good luck. He smiled but didn't say anything that morning, after arriving at the hospital, when he saw Dr. Nelson just before he was to perform the shunt procedure. The doctor wore a tie Teddi had given him for Christmas.

Teddi's head was prepped and then draped for the surgical procedure. Nelson then made an incision into the old scar. The incision went as far as the bone. Dr. Nelson then drilled a hole about a quarter of an inch in diameter into the skull. Almost immediately, fluid rushed out. It would drain for a full day.

After the procedure was over, it did seem that Teddi's coma lightened some. Tod was alone with her when she even opened up her eyes for a few moments. Tod told his sister that he loved her, and he also said good-bye to her.

Suctioning was now used to remove increasingly large amounts of green bile which was forming. Teddi's respiration then returned to being very labored. She even gurgled at times, as though she was trying to catch her breath. Because Teddi's improvement was minimal after two days had passed, Dr. Nelson recommended that the shunt be removed. The Mervises delayed a few days more because Sally Masten also reported that Teddi had opened her eyes.

Anne Cameron wrote "Happy Valentine's Day" on Teddi's medical chart. That day, the Mervises threw a pizza party for the children and staff on Teddi's floor. Sheri also made little bags of candy hearts and brought dozens of homemade cookies. After kidding Gary that they each wanted a dozen roses for Valentine's Day, they were delighted when Gary came to the party carrying a bouquet for each of them.

In those final days, Irene Matichyn brought her mother to the hospital. The woman wanted to see the child that called her "Baba"—which in Ukrainian meant "grandmother." After they left Teddi's room, Irene's mother started to cry. Irene told her: "If you break down I'll clobber you." In halting English, Baba looked up and said, "I no cry for Teddi. I cry for the mother."

Irene took her mother home and returned. Late that night, just she and Sheri were in the room. Sheri told her she sensed their friends were feeling guilty because while they loved Teddi, they were also glad it wasn't their child dying with a tumor. Irene felt her eyes welling up with tears. "I would be lying to you if I said I would rather it was my little girl lying there."

Meanwhile, Dr. Nelson was testing the medical waters for further consultation on his own. He called specialists at the University of Maryland to inquire about "hypothermia" as a possible treatment for Teddi. It was a relatively new technique of reducing tumors through the use of heat but specialists there would not recommend it in Teddi's case. Nelson also called Dr. Charles Wilson at the University of California Medical School in San Francisco. He asked his colleague there for his view about the possibility of further surgery on Teddi.

It was February 24th now and Teddi was still hanging on. Nurse Barb Fredette took her friend Anne Cameron aside that night, before switching shifts. She was becoming anxious, she said. The doctors didn't know why or how Teddi was staying alive. Did she, Anne, think there was much time left for Teddi? Barb wondered if it all could go on much longer.

The next afternoon, February 25th, with just Sheri in the room, Teddi cried out "Mama" several times. This unnerved Sheri, for no matter what she herself said or did, Teddi did not respond.

It was Friday, February 26th, at 4:30 P.M., and Polly Schwensen came by to see Teddi before going home. She was in good spirits for she told Sheri she just came from being with a mother who had lost her daughter to leukemia and the woman had remarkable faith and positiveness. She hoped that it would give Sheri hope.

Sheri listened, nodding her head. "Chuckie Altamara's mother came by this afternoon and said the same thing—'Don't worry, it will end. You'll wake up with this terrible ache in your heart in the middle of the night but call me. I don't care what time it is. Call me.' "

Sheri left Polly alone in the room while she went to make a phone call.

Polly moved her chair close to Teddi's bed, so she could be near her face. She stroked Teddi's head.

Near her ear, Polly told the child that it was the weekend and that she was going home from the hospital. She told Teddi she would miss her. She stroked Teddi's face, feeling odd about looking at someone, being almost able to examine them, and not have them know it. Polly saw Teddi's red stretch marks, the bloated face, the child's lack of hair, and her heart began to sink. But she reminded herself as well that there was still the spirit of a child in that body, and that spirit was still Teddi's. "I don't know if you can hear me," she whispered loudly, "but I'm going to say good-bye now. Good-bye, Teddi."

After Sheri returned, and saying good-bye to her as well, Polly ran into Dr. Nelson. She told him the Mervises were thinking of taking Teddi home. "What do you think about that?" she asked.

She saw feelings of loss and possibly love in his eyes. "I'd go along with that," he nodded, his voice soft.

Polly's heart was even more exuberant now. "A lot of people around here are bitching," she told herself, "but this guy has definitely been touched. The family taught him something."

Sheri noticed a change in Teddi that night. She told her brother-in-law Bob: "She looks more peaceful than in any other time of her stay." Bob, Sheri, and Gary left the hospital around midnight. Teddi's hospital record for those twenty-four hours closed with the words: "stable and comfortable."

Early the next morning—it was a Saturday—Teddi Mervis, a child whose brief life had touched the lives of so many others, died alone. Nothing heroic was attempted. The real heroism lay lifeless upon the bed.

29

Come Saturday Morning

Sheri and Gary were awakened that morning by the sound of the phone ringing. They knew what it was for even before answering. Afterward, they drove to the hospital together, just like they had so many times before, just like that first time, so long ago now, when they followed behind the ambulance thinking that maybe Teddi had had an epileptic seizure of some sort.

The policy at Strong Memorial Hospital is that nurses involved in primary care are notified even before coming to work if their patient dies. Said Anne, "It's sometimes easier to deal with it when you're at home." Anne got dressed and went to the hospital. Having arrived before the Mervises, she went into Teddi's room. Her eyes filled with tears. Teddi looked peaceful and Anne continued her prayers. "I know you're well now," she whispered, close to Teddi's face. "You've always been a special person to me." She leaned down and kissed Teddi for the last time.

Anne went to her desk to call Barb and Sally Masten. She got Barb on the phone first. When Barb heard Anne's voice she let out a small cry for she knew instantly what it was about.

"I don't have good news," Anne told her friend.

"It's Teddi, isn't it?" came Barb's reply.

All Anne then said was "yes," and Barb began to cry. Anne told her she would talk to her later.

Barb sat down at her kitchen table, her bathrobe on, and cried by herself that morning. Somehow, even though she knew it was coming, she still doubted, and wondered, and had not been fully emotionally prepared. The three nurses, Anne, Barb, and Sally, would say they all prayed especially for Gary that morning, because somehow they didn't believe he would ever be able to let go of his little girl.

Anne was still at her desk when the Mervises arrived. They went directly into Teddi's room. Anne called Dr. Nazarian and told him what had happened. She also talked to Sally. Anne waited for the Mervises to be alone with Teddi for some time before joining them.

She then got up slowly from her desk. She told herself not to cry. Anne stood in the back of Teddi's room for a few moments, deciding when it was appropriate for her to move forward. Gary and Sheri were both weeping and Anne slipped her arms around both of them and cried with them, too.

After some moments, Sheri asked Anne details of Teddi's death. "Were the agreed-upon procedures followed?" she wanted to know. Anne said she checked and they indeed had been. Sheri asked the nurse other questions, and Anne answered the best she could, aware all the time that Gary was sobbing and holding onto Teddi.

Dr. Nazarian entered the hospital corridor where Teddi's room was. He naturally didn't like these occasions, but he also felt that during times like these parents sometimes needed their doctor most. He thought to himself, to shore himself up, that Teddi was no longer suffering now. He also was appreciative of the fact that Teddi died at the hospital rather than at home, so the Mervises would not feel guilty that not all that medically could have been done was done. He entered the room without speaking and stayed with them without speaking. He took turns holding one and then the other Mervis, crying along with each of them.

Anne called Polly to tell her of Teddi's death. At first Polly felt relieved. Everything had worked out, she thought—her conversation with Sheri, the prayers Teddi wouldn't die on Anne's shift, all that and so much more. But then, on a walk by herself, she came across the morning paper. Its headline read: "12-year-old Teddi Mervis Dies of Brain Tumor." Polly bought the paper and stood there in the snow reading further down the page. She lingered with a quote by Gary.

"No matter how you plan," he had said, "it was still something to have that warm body there. You could talk to her—and whether she could hear us or not in the last few weeks, we don't know. But you could hug her and squeeze her—and now she's gone." It was then, for the first time that morning, she began to cry, on the cold city street, by herself.

All Irene Matichyn had to say on the phone that morning was "Skipper, honey" and Skip knew instantly Teddi had died. Irene said Gary and Sheri were heading home now. Skip hung up the phone and turned around. His wife stood there. Cheryl lowered her eyes and left the room.

As Skip drove to the Mervis home he talked out loud. He remembered later saying "all those macho things" he had learned along the way. "I don't know what we're going to find when we get there and I don't know what kind of an ordeal this is going to be, but God knows it can't be any worse than the ordeal that they've gone through." He looked over at his wife and then back to the road. "But somebody's got to be strong. Let Gary not be—and Sheri not be. You will be and I will be."

Cheryl was half-listening, knowing her husband was trying to strengthen himself for the ordeal ahead. She still felt in shock from the news of Teddi's death. As Skip pulled into the driveway she panicked for a moment, suddenly thinking maybe they shouldn't have come, that maybe the Mervises would want to be alone. "I don't care," Cheryl said to herself. "I really don't care. I need to be with them. They may not need me but I need them."

Betty Scobell, next-door neighbor to the Mervises, called the hospital each day to find out how Teddi was doing. That morning a neighbor from across the street called her. "Is everything all right with the Mervises?" she asked, knowing that Betty was a good friend of the family.

"I don't know," Betty answered. She hesitated, "Why do you ask?"

"I saw the Mervises leave about quarter to seven," said the neighbor.

Betty Scobell called the hospital and got the news that way. She watched as the cars pulled into the driveway next door and were to park up and down the street throughout the day. She would wait, she thought, until Sheri and Gary were alone before she and her husband Jim would pay their respects, too.

When Irene Matichyn arrived at the Mervis home she tried to appear confident and strong. Tod and Kim were watching TV; Sheri was in the bedroom. Gary looked up and Irene went over and kissed him. "I'm going to make some coffee," she said, "and look—I've got some of your favorite doughnuts."

Sheri entered and Irene kissed her. "I'm sorry, honey," she told Sheri. "What can I do? I'm here to cook. To clean. What do you want me to do?"

They sat down and had coffee together in the kitchen. Irene tried to keep the conversation up, like a balloon in the air, but Sheri started to unravel that morning's events, how the phone call had come, how they went into her hospital room to touch Teddi.

Irene nodded but would have a difficult time remembering the conversation. All her energies, she said, were focused on not breaking down in front of Sheri. Irene would have felt too guilty afterward, she said, showing her pain after what a mother had endured. One piece of the conversation did stay with Irene and that was when Sheri said she didn't think Gary really believed Teddi was dead until he saw her. Then he held onto her and cried and wouldn't let go.

On the surface, Tod and Kim appeared to be taking the news well. Later, Kim would say that that morning and the mornings which soon followed seemed like a dream to her. She knew what was happening, and she talked and listened and even cried, but somehow she remained detached from it all.

Tod also held up well thus far. The morning of Teddi's death he had a question for his mother. "Mom—," he said, "do you think it will be all right if I were one of Teddi's pallbearers?"

Sheri nodded her assent but wondered how he had learned about such things, never having gone to a funeral himself. Tod, however, had seen a funeral in a movie and learned that the people who carried the casket were considered to be very dear to the person who died.

Sheri was taking a shower when the DeBiases arrived. Cheryl took Kim and Tod into the kitchen so Skip could be alone with Gary. Skip went to where Gary was sitting, took his hand and kneeled next to him.

Gary looked into Skip's eyes and started sobbing.

"Gary," Skip was saying, "she was strong."

"She was, wasn't she?" Gary said, biting his lip.

Skip nodded his support. "She certainly was a fighter."

Gary started to cry again. "But she couldn't beat it. She didn't beat it, did she?"

Skip squeezed his hand. "Listen, Gary, she made life a lot more worth living for a lot of people."

Sheri then entered the room. Cheryl, hearing her, was in the doorway. Cheryl remembered that she looked calm, though knew her well enough to understand her heart was broken inside.

Anne Cameron came by after her shift with some of Teddi's personal effects, and a paperback book Gary had left at the hospital. Gary said he had something for her and left. When he came back he gave Anne a stickpin which said "The Teddi Award." It was a kind of Camp medal for valor in the fight against cancer above and beyond the call of duty. "If anybody deserves this award," he said, "you do."

Phones rang elsewhere throughout the city and beyond, carrying word that the beloved Teddi Mervis had died. Laurie Allinger stopped crying long enough to call Suzie Parker and started crying all over again.

"What are we going to do without Teddi," she told Suzie Parker. "What are we going to do at Camp without her?"

"We'll do what we always do," Suzie exclaimed. "We'll carry on."

That was the first time Laurie Allinger wondered if there would be a Camp the following year, now that Teddi had died. She wondered if there would even be a Teddi Project any more now that the inspiration for it all was gone.

Muggs Register, in her dorm room at Geneseo College, felt defeated when she hung up the phone that morning. On the drive back to Rochester her thoughts turned to Camp and to the time she huddled next to the deaf and nearly blind child on the floor at the Camp Christmas party. The long drive back to Rochester wasn't long enough to hold all the memories Muggs had with Teddi.

Drs. Omar Salazar and Martin Klemperer were no longer in Rochester but were called and told of Teddi's death. They were naturally sad, but also relieved, that Teddi's terrible pain was at an end and the strain on her parents and friends was also over. They would write to the Mervises, trying to console from long distance.

Dr. Nazarian came by the Mervis house that day as well. He sat at the table with Sheri and Gary and talked about Teddi, her personality, and her great courage. The talk turned to religion, and Dr. Nazarian, a physician with faith, shared his deep-seated belief that he thought this life was a prelude to the next and a better one. "Somebody like Teddi," he said, "has moved onto another realm. The more living and working I do," he added, "the stronger my faith becomes."

Though he had faith, he still believed in using the optimum that medical science and technologies had to offer. Though he had faith, he never forced it upon others—and yet neither did he feel it inappropriate to talk about it when asked.

Father Ambuske came. They talked about Teddi some more, and more laughter returned to the Mervis home. The priest told them about the time Teddi had cautioned him about wearing his brown suit too often, and about her request that "Sweet'Ums" the bulldog be in the room in their more private conversations.

He told them, before he left that afternoon, that Teddi had pretty much planned most of her own funeral. This surprised and in some ways saddened the Mervises. Ambuske, explaining some of the major points of the ceremony, asked if it would be all right if he proceeded according to her wishes. Both Mervises nodded their approval.

"There's one more thing," Father Ambuske said before leaving that day, "we'll need a bigger church. I don't think my church will be able to accommodate the number of people who will probably come."

After Father Ambuske left, Sheri left Gary to the newcomers, arriving almost by the minute now, to go and make arrangements for Teddi's coffin and burial. Deep down she also knew that as tough and scrappy as her husband was, matters such as this would crush him.

Sheri met with Mike Falvo, the newest son to enter his father's undertaking business. This funeral and family were special to Mike. He had been a counselor that previous summer at Camp. Later, Mike would recall how strong and direct Sheri was on that visit.

"No embalming," she told him. "Her body has been tampered with enough." She also told Mike she wanted Teddi to have "a simple wooden coffin so that it would decompose as quickly as possible along with Teddi's body." Sheri hesitated, "Her soul is with God now."

After that, she told Mike she wanted to have the "wake" for only one day, and that she wanted a closed casket. She wanted a stand by the casket, and on it she wanted Mike to put Teddietta, Teddi's beloved bear, and a letter Teddi had written to her Dad that Father's Day. Sheri said the letter would be framed and ready for Mike as soon as possible.

"What do you want to do about the wedding band?" Mike asked.

Teddi had taken Gary's wedding ring off one day and had never given it back. She never offered any explanation and Gary had let her keep it. Sheri told Mike to leave it in the casket with Teddi. "Tod wants to put this in with her, too," Sheri said, handing over her son's St. Michael's medal. St. Michael was the patron saint of the "underdog."

30

"Don't Hang onto Good-Bye"

There were only a dozen or so simple bouquets around and above Teddi's casket. Instead of flowers, people had begun making contributions to Camp Good Days and Special Times itself. The Camp was not about death, but life, and the donations from this and other funerals to follow would reflect people's changing attitudes toward children with cancer.

People began to trickle in. Nurses Barb Fredette and Anne Cameron arrived early and together. They saw Sheri and Gary and were unable to speak. They hugged Gary. Sheri returned with some tissues. "Here," she said, handing them over, "you'll probably need these this afternoon." Nurse Sally Masten arrived shortly thereafter. Angry with God, she was praying to her father and to fiance John as she approached the Mervises. "Take care of Teddi for us," she was praying inside. When she reached the Mervises she stuck out her hand to Gary. "I hope you know that I know what you're going through and just know that I love you, Teddi and Sheri."

Gary was crying. "We love all you guys," he was saying, "and we don't know what we would have done without you."

Polly Schwensen arrived. She was thinking about what had happened that day at work. A doctor had come up to her and said, "Did you see the papers where Mr. Mervis thought Teddi could still hear him in there?" Too angry to speak, Polly turned and walked away from the doctor. But now Polly was warmed by the fact that throughout the afternoon and evening Gary, though preoccupied with others, would ask her to stay close by. He would come over to talk to her whenever there was a break from the crowd of people that came into the funeral home.

The nurses, Polly Schwensen, and even some of the doctors felt compelled to attend the wakes and funerals of children they had helped care for. They had learned, from hard experience, that it was easier in the long run to come than to stay away. Seeing the children physically leave the earth and struggling through the sorrow along with the family and others they had come to hold dear brought each story to a close so that a new chapter was able to begin.

Of the process Polly would later say: "It's my way of knowing that they're really gone. Otherwise I'd think in my heart they were still all out there."

Betty Scobell and then Irene Matichyn arrived. Betty, carrying her own cancer, waited with her husband Jim to shake Gary's hand. "She's gone," Gary told her.

Betty had tears in her shiny blue eyes. "Maybe we can't see her but she'll never be gone, Gary,"

Irene Matichyn hugged Gary, trying to console him. Irene refused to cry. She turned to Sheri. "I'm so glad you didn't wear black," she said. "Teddi would just love the way you look. Teddi always liked it when you looked beautiful and you do." Irene didn't go to the coffin to pray, but instead worked her way to the back of the room to talk and to watch.

Mike Falvo, the young funeral director who had been at Camp, spotted Muggs Register and came over to talk to her. Muggs had noticed how hard he seemed to be trying, that he really looked concerned about the job he was doing. "I don't know if this is the best time to tell you this," he said to Muggs, and then unraveled a story about a close friend of his who was just diagnosed as having Hodgkin's disease. His friend was very depressed and afraid. "Sure," said Muggs, when he had finished, "I'll be glad to talk with her." Mike left and Muggs thought to herself, "Teddi's gone but it's not over. There are still a lot of other people to worry about."

Skip DeBiase was watching. He was stunned at the number of people who had come: powerful politicians, lawyers, doctors; men who came in their police uniforms and women who came from work with briefcases. Father Ambuske came to comfort and console, and because he is the kind of priest he is, he allowed others to comfort and console him as well. Camp counselors arrived in groups of twos and threes, and alone. Mike and Jim Menz, two strong, gentle brothers who had such a good time with the kids at Camp that somebody had remarked they ought to be charged for going, felt as though they had lost a sister. It was a bitter cold day and yet the large funeral home was overflowing with mourners.

And then Skip watched as the children from Camp arrived, all together and with nervous looks on their faces. The crowd grew quiet and parted, allowing them to reach the Mervises and Teddi's coffin. As if there had not been enough sadness and tears, the sight of these small soldiers—with amputated limbs, walking with canes and crutches, faces pale and sometimes wearing wigs—made some, such as Skip, gasp for their next breath. "Life doesn't get much harder than this," Skip thought to himself. He knew what was on their minds. Camp had brought them together and these children now unequivocally knew, as Laurie Allinger would say afterward, that they were all "going to see a lot of death now."

Afterward, after the Camp kids had passed by the coffin, Skip and a few of the counselors got them together in an adjoining room. They were sad at first but lightened up some with Skip's stories about fishing hooks getting caught in the trees and spaghetti being served up as worms to blind-folded nurses. "Blasphemy," he said, shaking his head, " using spaghetti that way." Skip noted that nearly every child with cancer who left that night said they were really going to miss Teddi. He thought it the greatest of tributes, coming from Teddi's own peers.

Sheri, throughout the wake, continued to make final arrangements for Teddi. She saw Karen Lenio and took her aside. "Your son's picture is in there with Teddi," she said, nodding with her head in the direction of the casket. Eric Lenio had sometimes come with his mother to see Teddi. "Teddi liked him very much," Sheri said.

Cheryl DeBiase was about to leave the funeral home when Sheri stopped her. "Being so close to Teddi," Sheri said, "is there anything you'd like to put in there with her?"

Cheryl thought for a moment. "How about Teddietta? Are you going to put her in there?"

Sheri shook her head. She couldn't let go of Teddietta too.

"Well, Teddi will need a stuffed animal with her," Cheryl said. She left and came back with a stuffed donkey she had bought for Teddi. It was a symbol for her. "When you were stubborn you were stubborn," she said, thinking about the hard and endearing times when Teddi's strong will showed itself. The stuffed donkey along with letters from each member of the DeBiase family were to be buried along with Teddi.

Cheryl DeBiase would have a hard time sleeping that night. The funeral was the next morning and she tossed and turned what seemed the entire night. As soon as she fell into a deep sleep she would shake herself awake, afraid she would miss the funeral. It seemed to take forever for morning to come.

Her husband Skip, looking in the mirror that morning while shaving, stopped and lingered, trying to remember what his face looked like when he had his first turn at being a pallbearer. His eldest son was to be a pallbearer that morning for Teddi and he wanted to try and remember what he had felt like, years and dozens of funerals before.

Irene, finishing dressing, was wondering whether she should wear her false eyelashes that morning. She had not cried since Teddi died. She was glad, at that point in the day anyway, that Teddi was no longer in pain. Many a night she had driven home from the hospital saying, "When is it going to end? Godamnit, this is enough." Irene put on her eyelashes feeling hard and angry inside.

Laurie Allinger was ready that morning long before her ride was supposed to arrive. Laurie was afraid she would "do something stupid" at the funeral and embarrass herself and the other people there. When one of her grandparents had died, a few years before, she laughed throughout the entire funeral service. "If I get stupid just bop me on the head," she told the person driving her that morning.

Barb Fredette and Anne Cameron arrived about twenty minutes before the funeral was to start and were lucky to find a seat even then. The large church was nearly filled, and soon others began to set up folding chairs in the aisles and back. The line would extend, once the funeral started, down the church's front steps and onto the street.

Barb looked around and saw a lot of kids from Camp there. Some saw her and tried to smile, a few even waved. It made Barb cry, thinking that Teddi had brought so many wonderful people together. Friend Anne Cameron is not the type of person to cry in public. But when she got a glimpse of the sad way both Gary and Sheri looked she leaned against her dear friend Barb with her hurting heart.

Sally Masten was having a miserable time inside, waiting for the funeral to start. Unlike many of the others, she was not glad Teddi's suffering was over—she was angry that it had to start at all. Her old pain returned, and she almost got up to leave. Polly Schwensen, an Episcopalian, felt good being in an Episcopal Church. Then she got a glimpse of Kim, sitting in an aisle seat next to the casket, and she suddenly burst into tears. She could deal with almost anything except watching children having to struggle with this.

Dr. Nazarian was also in attendance. He juggled his busy schedule and sat there hoping the Mervises were feeling his conviction that Teddi was in a better, nicer place. He also began to hurt some for the family, too, knowing of the pain. And then he hurt for himself, realizing he was going to miss Teddi, who had become his friend.

Skip DeBiase sat near the Mervises, fuming inside. He was upset because a television crew had come in and was setting up its cameras. He thought it an unbelievable intrusion into a private moment and felt himself start to get up. He waited, instead, to see if Gary was going to give him a cue to throw them out. When none came, he turned his thoughts inward. For some reason he couldn't stop going over the words from "The Rainbow Connection." He didn't cry, though, until he saw his son walk down the aisle as a pallbearer. He wanted to get up and leave but his wife and three children were beside him and he stayed for them, knowing they would want him to, and that if he left they might not be able to emotionally hang on themselves. Skip would later say he knew a good eulogy was given, because so many commented about it, but he never could recall a single word for himself.

Cheryl DeBiase held onto the hand of their six-year-old daughter. That morning the child insisted she be allowed to go to the funeral, too. "I gotta do my respects," she had said. "Teddi was my friend too."

Cheryl saw the pallbearers come, all young, all handsome, including her own son who had flirted with Teddi so many times, telling her he was going to be her first date. "Boy," Cheryl thought to herself, "I bet you feel like a big wheel now with all these big, strong boys around you."

Barb Fredette, who had stopped crying, fell into deeper sorrow when Tod passed her by. "He was trying to be a brave boy," she remembered. Laurie Allinger was experiencing all kinds of strange sensations and delusions at the funeral. For one thing, she kept imagining monsters coming out of Teddi's casket. She would remember Tod going by, carrying his sister. "He sort of looked at me like—'Don't cry'—because I was crying so hard. But I couldn't stop no matter what anybody said or did."

Anne Kiefer caught a glimpse of Gary's face as he turned toward Sheri, and in that instance she realized the separation was going to be real now. She started to cry, and, sensing somebody from behind was watching her, turned to see a child from her cabin at Camp. The child was crying but extended her hand to Anne, who held on to it throughout the service.

Not all of the Mervis's many friends, or those who had become associated with Camp Good Days and Special Times, came to the wake or the funeral. Some people couldn't, or wouldn't deal with it, and drifted away, not stopping by, calling or writing to extend their condolences, never acknowledging their relationship with the Mervises or the Camp again.

It was a very simple service that morning, almost stark. Beginning with a few brief prayers on behalf of Teddi's soul, Father Dave Ambuske then took some of the notes he had made for himself to the pulpit with him. He paused. He could hear the wind blowing outside, and the muffled sounds of people crying and comforting one another inside.

He said a small prayer for himself, and to Teddi, asking for her help and for the courage, as he had promised, not to cry. "Oh God," he intoned, "whose beloved Son did take little children into his arms and bless them: Give us grace, we beseech thee, to entrust this child Elizabeth to thy never-failing care and love..."

Ambuske felt his heart begin to pound and paused, just like it was something he was supposed to do, and in that pause he took in the huge crowd that had gathered, the powerful and small children, mothers and fathers and a host of friends. He thought of Teddi saying she hoped her life had been symbolized in the picture of God touching Adam's finger in the Sistine Chapel—that she had touched that many people. Ambuske fought back the desire to cry, recognizing that she had indeed touched hundreds of hearts.

He began by telling those gathered that "Teddi Mervis asked me some of the most difficult questions I've ever been asked."

... I told her, when she asked to be baptized, that she would now be a child of God. But then she wanted to know if there were other children of God and

I told her yes, and some didn't have a priest or rabbi to be with them, but if they did the right thing then they were children of God, too.

"Teddi said," and with this Ambuske brought scattered chuckles from the crowd, ". . . Teddi wanted to know why, if there were so many children of God, there was so much trouble in the world too!"

Ambuske continued, telling them that Teddi had said that if all religions were supposed to love one another, then why didn't they? He said she had often made him answer with words like "mystery" and "faith" and that he didn't know all the answers to her questions.

" 'I'll probably know some of these answers before you will, won't I, Dave?' she had said, and I told her she probably would."

He told some of the other things she had said and realized, at that point, that he was no longer referring to his notes. He was talking with the same ease, and peace, he had had when talking to Teddi alone. And the priest went on to tell them other things. "She was looking forward to meeting God. I told her that there will be others in heaven she knew, like the boys and girls from Camp. I told her I didn't know how they were going to communicate but that I definitely believed they were. 'It will be a lot like earth, Teddi,' I had said, 'except there won't be any tears.' "

"Teddi nodded then," the priest said, "and she would say, after a while, that 'tears were bad.' "

Lest those who listened thought Teddi didn't spiritually hurt, he told them of the times when her sadness and anger returned to her, asking the priest why she had been selected out to suffer so. She wanted to live, she said, live a long life, become a teacher, do things that so many other kids her age were going to get to do.

"But in time," Ambuske said, nearing the finish of what he wanted to say, "Teddi Mervis came to grips with her fate, just as she had with her terrible disease. We talked about suffering and its meaning. And together we came to the idea that suffering is only meaningless if we can't find its purpose. We talked about Camp and all the kids who were now able to enjoy life a little because of it. Toward the end," the priest said, "Teddi said to me—'I must have been chosen. I must have been meant to do something on earth. Why not me, right Dave? That's what I should be saying.' "

His own feelings of loss were starting to fill him now, and he found himself saying: "She told me—'Make it happy, Dave. I'm just leaving one side and going to another. It's not good-bye, that's not what I'm doing, I'm saying 'hello.' Tell them not to hang onto good-byes, that I don't like good-byes.' "

Before turning from the pulpit Father Ambuske remembered the message Gary had passed onto him, to invite all those present to the Mervis home after the burial.

The priest, and all those present, sat in silence for a few moments. Cheryl Debiase was very grateful that Father Ambuske stopped when he did, she didn't feel she could take anymore. Bob Mervis seldom cries but he did then. He had seen Ambuske at the hospital, had watched his face. He knew Ambuske spoke from the heart. Nurse Barb Fredette remembered it as being a happy sermon but that was about all. She could picture Teddi talking the way she had to the priest. Anne Cameron felt proud afterward that she had come to know somebody so good. Teacher Karen Lenio wanted more, she wanted this eulogy to be "cataclysmic and cathartic." She said she wanted it to be "perfect."

The hearts of others took different turns in the listening and silence which followed. Irene Matichyn was crying hard as the eulogy ended. What the priest had said was truly the Teddi she had known. "So up, so cheery," thought Irene. "And so opposite of me the cynic." Sande Macaluso was standing in the back of the church feeling his heart hardened. "How could we have spent millions—maybe billions—going to the moon," he was thinking to himself, "and we could not save the single life of this wonderful child."

Gary and Sheri walked side by side directly behind the casket as it was being wheeled from the church. Irene would remember how Sheri's face looked. "The haunting expression, the sunken eyes," said Irene. "She wasn't crying but I go back to my own religious upbringing, being raised Catholic, and I think of how the Blessed Mother would have felt and looked the day her Son was crucified. . . . You could see the devastation on that mother's face." When the Mervises passed by her pew, Polly Schwensen thought of President Kennedy's funeral.

Muggs Register watched, strong and without tears, as the procession passed. She was doing all right until some of the children from Camp passed her pew—Laurie Allinger, Mark Dillon, more faces she had come to know and love—and Muggs sat back down in her pew, burying her face in her hands, crying. She thought afterward she was crying for the children, for what they had to endure themselves, and for what they had to take on, too, in the death of friends.

The long train of cars left the church for the cemetery a few miles away. The February wind blew cruel and crazy, as people exited their cars and walked the small icy road to the grave site. Some of Teddi's fellow campers needed help along the way. So did some of the older women and the men who cried.

Father Ambuske said but a few words because of the blustery cold. He was surprised so many had come, right to the bitter end, as if they were protesting heaven itself for taking one of earth's littlest and best.

Sally Masten remembers Sheri with her arm around Gary. Skip, standing behind the Mervises, caught a glimpse of his son, standing near the casket, tears frozen on his face. "He'll have to go through this alone now," Skip thought to himself. "I can't do anything for him now."

Cheryl DeBiase, on the fringe of the crowd, stood with her six-year-old daughter. The child had difficulty making it to the burial site but had refused to turn back. Cheryl, helping her, tried to make herself happy with thoughts of Teddi no longer having cancer, and being taken care of by Gary's mother, and finding old friend Chuckie Altamara. But selfish thoughts took over at the end, when people put a carnation on Teddi's casket and whispered prayers of good-bye. "I don't care if she is sick," thought Cheryl. "I want her back."

A sudden shudder went through Barb Fredette that she knew wasn't from the cold. "This is indeed the end," she thought to herself. No more tears would come for her now. Betty Scobell could see Tod. She smiled. God how she liked him. "He's such a 'Dennis the Menace'," she would say. "But he's so grown up today." She didn't remember seeing tears in Tod's eyes at the wake or at the funeral service. But as he left his sister, Betty saw him sobbing. A pain deeper than her repeated surgeries registered inside her. She gripped her husband's arm.

Uppermost in Tod's mind that morning was doing his job. The sidewalk to the church was narrow, and on his side of the casket they walked mostly in the snow. They almost slipped once. He tried to be brave, as others remembered, in the church and walking down the aisle. Only now, with his work at an end, would Tod release the sorrow inside.

Skip DeBiase was one of the last to leave. He put a carnation on Teddi's casket, whispering, "I love you comare." Father Ambuske, putting his flower on the tomb of his friend, wanted to know if she was going to allow him to cry now.

Two people hung back from the crowd that bitter morning. One was Muggs Register. She felt she had a special relationship with her departed friend that couldn't be acknowledged with so many people around. Muggs found it hard to communicate and pray being distracted by the souls of so many. She wouldn't notice Polly, who also waited behind, and who also wanted a few moments alone with Teddi before her physical presence would be gone from this earth forever. "It's just like always," Polly thought to herself. "Always too many people around you. They never seem to give me a chance. I couldn't even see the ceremony." And then Polly stopped herself, put a smile on her face, knew that the important thing was that Teddi would be with God now. "Good-bye," she whispered, "see you later."

Walking down the hill, Polly saw Laurie Allinger walking alone, head down. She caught up with Laurie and put an arm around the teen-ager. Polly noticed others were hesitant to do this because Laurie had no arm.

"How are you doing with all this?" Polly asked.

Laurie said she rode horseback hard the night before to relieve herself of some of the pain. They talked a little more, Laurie never mentioning that she had only gotten halfway up the hill and had turned back, not being able to see it all through to the very end.

Not everyone went to the ceremony that morning. Anne Kiefer, Teddi's first counselor, went home instead and wrote a letter to some people she had met on vacation. They had been curious about Camp Good Days and Special Times and now Anne told them all they needed to know, and she told them personally and from the bottom of her heart. They would respond with a large donation to the Camp.

31

A Dreadful Silence

Sheri reached the front door of her house and stopped suddenly. Bob Mervis was on one side of her, his wife Linda on the other. Now, for the first time throughout the ordeal of the wake, funeral, and cemetery service, Sheri broke down. "I think I'm going to throw up," she said. She trembled: this was home and the first step into it without Teddi.

Linda asked if she wanted to go some place else for a while.

"No, I'll be okay," Sheri said, and took a deep breath and went inside.

Inside, close friends were already preparing food for the large crowd that would arrive. Commotion reigned, and one could hear people beginning to joke with each other. "Hey, who cooked this?" somebody would ask. "This is terrible," another person would say.

Throughout the rest of the day and evening Sheri walked around the room making sure everybody had something to eat and that they were comfortable, and all the while she held Teddietta close to her, in the middle of her chest, over her heart.

Skip noticed that Gary seemed to be withdrawn. The house had become very hot and stuffy at this point, with the crowd of people that had jammed in. "Come walk with me," Skip told him, taking Gary's hand.

Once outside, wearing only their sports coats, the two walked up and down the street. At first the old questions returned to Gary, the ones beginning with "why." Then Gary began to express his disbelief in it all—Teddi getting a tumor, what she had gone through, the fact that she was gone. "I don't know what to do with my life now," he told Skip. "Teddi has been so much of my life. So much of my energies have been devoted there."

He told Skip that after the wake he had gone to the grocery store to pick up a few things and found he had bought a jar of Teddi's favorite marmalade.

The morning of the funeral, after pulling out of the driveway, he had headed in the direction of the hospital and not the church.

Gary seemed relieved after they had talked some and said he wanted to go back inside. They both marveled at the number of cars in the driveway and on both sides of the road up and down the street where they had walked.

Teddi's three nurses, Barb, Anne, and Sally, came in and greeted Gary. The three had debated whether or not to go to the Mervis house after the graveside ceremony. It would be crowded, they wouldn't know many of the people there, and deep down they weren't sure if Gary and Sheri were really pleased with the quality of care they had tried to give Teddi.

Gary sat with the three of them for a long while at the kitchen table. The attention he paid them showed how much he respected what they had done and how close he felt to them. Afterward, Barb thought that Gary and Sheri felt close to the three of them because they were the only ones, other than themselves, who saw Teddi day in and day out for the duration of her ordeal.

Before the three left that day, Gary said he had something he wanted to find. He left the room and didn't return for quite some time and they, like Sheri, had become anxious. But Gary came back smiling, saying he was losing his memory, and couldn't remember where he had left two more "Teddi Award" stickpins. Anne already had one and he now gave the other two to Barb and Sally. "I know Teddi would want you both to have it for being so brave," he told them.

The three said their good-byes, with Sally Masten going last. Sally would later recall that Gary's face looked especially worn, "like he could cry at the drop of a hat." Though angry with God sometimes for the fate she herself had been delivered, Sally left that day a little lighter in her heart, knowing that while all people may share suffering and death, on the human plane they also share love. When Barb Fredette said her prayers that night, she asked God to watch over the Mervises and to take care of Teddi.

Anne Cameron felt stronger from her experience with Teddi. "If that little girl could be so brave," she said, "then I can be more brave, too." Just as a reminder of the source of her courage, nurse Anne Cameron wears the "Teddi Award" on the collar of her uniform each day at work. She would also say, afterward, how much she missed the children she had taken care of and who had died, including Teddi. The one thing that kept her going was her belief that when it was her turn to go over to the other side, they would all be clapping and cheering to see her.

Irene Matichyn remained angry afterward, saying that, "If I was the guy designing the whole thing, with the universe and humanity, there is no way I would do it this way." She couldn't be convinced that there was any meaning to Teddi's death. "Teddi was a beautiful human being, a kind human being," Irene said, "and had she lived she would have made people happy."

The DeBiases stayed until nearly everyone else was gone. Skip was at the table with Gary. He told Gary, as his farewell for the day: "This has been a hard day. But this is when the day gets the hardest. Now it's you and the family—and the loss is going to have to be dealt with." He gave Gary a hug before he left, saying, "I just hope to God that you're all so exhausted you'll just go and pass out."

Skip and Cheryl put their children to bed, and then Cheryl lay down on the couch and quickly fell asleep. She was completely drained and also at peace. She was remembering the time, before Teddi had gone into a coma, when she told Cheryl: " I love my mommy and daddy but if they weren't here I'd have you." Not always confident in herself, Cheryl also was grateful that she had been strong when she needed to be. Teddi had left her that, too, along with love.

His wife and children asleep, and the long ordeal at an end, Skip was nervous. He didn't know what to do with himself now. And so he paced, later taking a bottle of scotch from the liquor cabinet with him. He left a note for Cheryl: "Don't worry. I need to be alone for a while."

Then Skip drove around the city for awhile, the scotch still in its bottle, for some reason ending up near the airport. He thought about that afterward, if somehow his driving there meant he wanted to leave—at least for a while— the burden that he saw people carrying. He pulled into the Sheraton Hotel, across the road from the airport and rented a room. He drank two glasses of scotch. And then the man who stood by Gary, sang with Teddi, held up Irene, remained strong for his family, and showed the world that a lake lived, let his heart finally do what it had been aching to do for three years. He raised his glass saying "salude comare," and then he cried.

On the other side of the city, Father Dave Ambuske was winding his alarm clock. He could see out the window that the wind had died down. It looked calm outside now, though awfully cold. "Finally you are at rest," he said, turning out the light. And as he lay there on the pillow he smiled a little, knowing that Teddi had all her answers now.

Later, when the priest consoled those who were seriously ill and their loved ones, he would sometimes draw upon his experience with Teddi, telling others about the child's courage, saying they could pray to her for help.

Laurie Allinger tossed and turned that night. She thought about Teddi in the context of the "blood sisters." Where they were once four, now they were down to three. Would they end up with two and then one? Then maybe nobody at all would be left? She cried herself to sleep, remembering saying to Teddi—"I wish you didn't have to go. I'll go and trade you for me so you can live and I can die. You were more special—with the Camp and all— than me."

When Laurie went to school the following morning her classmates told her they saw the funeral on television with their parents, and people were crying. Toughened by the experience, Laurie also changed her attitude about herself. "I grew up a lot," she would later say. "And now when people ask me where's my arm I tell 'em I left it at home—that I didn't need it that particular day."

Polly Schwensen wanted badly to go to the Mervis house after the cemetary service but had to go back to work. After work she had a church supper to go to. Still, she said she felt something akin to being "unfinished." It was then she had one of those little talks with herself. "You're always withdrawing," she thought. "Now you get out there and go over and see the Mervises and tell them you wanted to be there."

She wrote a personal note on a card she bought for the Mervis family and on the way over stopped and bought some apples. "They probably had too much starch all day," she thought, "and so I'll bring them some fruit."

She rang the doorbell of the Mervis home and as she stood there waiting, the card and the bag of apples in her arms, she started to panic. "This is dumb," she thought. "This is silly. It's nine o'clock and they're probably tired and already in bed and nobody else is here."

But then Gary answered the door. He smiled, clearly glad to see her.

"I just wanted you to know that I couldn't come earlier," Polly blurted, sounding like she was reading from a prepared text. "This is the end of my day and the first chance I've had to come over and see you."

Welcoming her inside, he thought of what Dr. Royer had said about social workers, and what he himself had believed. How he had come to love this woman of simple honesty and a caring heart.

Polly sprawled onto the floor with Sheri, while Gary sat in his favorite chair. They reminisced for a while, and toward the end of their conversation, Polly reminded them about the visit of the little boy whose name was Jesus. Polly felt that was an important thing for the family to remember. Though Kim and Tod were watching television nearby, and apparently not listening, Tod would later say that Polly's remarks about the little boy meant a lot to him. "I knew my sister was all right then," he later said.

Polly wanted to know what Gary was going to do the next day. "I'm going to sit in a hot tub all day," Gary said, smiling. And they all laughed.

"And what are you going to do the day after that?" she asked.

"The same thing!" Gary told her.

As she drove home that night, Polly was happy she had gone to see the Mervises. She felt complete now. And she thought to herself that if Teddi could get up in front of those TV cameras, and if Sheri—who Polly thought was extremely quiet and shy—could take charge of running the day-to-day details of a large Camp, then gosh darn it maybe she herself could show a little more courage now.

Kim Mervis would have a difficult time afterward. Saddened that maybe she could have been nicer to her sister, she also knew her life would never be the same. Tod Mervis said his prayers that night and afterwards remembered what his father had told him over the years—to remember the good and the bad each night and the next day try to improve upon the bad. Before falling asleep, he asked God "to please take care of my sister."

Tod would go to the cemetery often after that. When spring came he thought Teddi's place in the cemetery was a good one for it got a lot of sun. Each time he went, as is the custom of the Jews, he placed a stone on Teddi's grave, a reminder to others that someone had been there.

Afterward, for Gary and Sheri, there would be this terrible silence—a dreadful deafening silence. How they ached to hear Teddi's voice, to have her questions again, even the hard ones with no answers. They strained to hear sometimes, especially at night when the house was quiet. Sometimes the floors creaked and they thought she was up; sometimes they walked into her bedroom forgetting.

Teddi's birthday, the start of school, Christmas, all lay ahead and would have to be endured. Maybe after that, after a full year had passed, Teddi would be able to come back again, only this time to a different place in the heart.

32

To Go on Anyway

The spring after Teddi died, until early summer, people associated with Camp Good Days and Special Times, especially the children with cancer, had just one question on their minds: would Camp continue now that its main inspiration, Teddi Mervis, was dead? They wondered, too, if that third camping season would be it. Would Camp organizers give them one more shot at a summer camping experience and then it would be over? Give it up for good? Still others wondered if the third camp would be so sad and so depressing it would have been a good idea not to have it at all; that nobody would even want to come back another year.

For all intents and purposes, that third summer would be crucial not only to the children with cancer but to the long-term survival of Camp Good Days and Special Times. Campers and counselors *had* to come back. They had to endure the loss of Teddi, and others who had died throughout the year, and learn to go on anyway. They would have to all learn now and for sure that it wasn't how much time they had left but what they did with it that mattered.

The night before the campers arrived, Gary Mervis rose to speak. Those who knew him thought he was different, and they glanced at each other around and across tables to see if others could tell. "You counselors are the ones who make it work now," he said. "You get to know the kids on a one-to-one basis. You're there at night when they want someone to talk to. You've got a special mission to give the children a week they'll never forget."

All listened intently, including Skip, respecting the difficulty Gary was experiencing. He continued, looking down, leaning on his hand: "We lost twenty-one children in two years, and seventeen of them since the last Camp." Finishing, Gary said he expected two things of them all: "Send them home happy. And send them home safe."

Those sitting next to Skip felt him move, ever so slightly. He felt an urge to rise and speak, but didn't know how his words might affect the Mervises. What Skip wanted to say was that not a single kid had died, not really—that the spirit of each one of those children was there in the Camp. But Skip hesitated, and then let it pass, as others would let other things pass that week. They would try to make the best of it, with the Mervis sorrow on one hand, and the desire to give the children as much joy and tender giving as possible on the other. Skip knew, and the others soon would also, that Gary's father had died just before Camp was to open. And so in six months the man who had founded Camp Good Days and Special Times had lost both the oldest and the youngest in his family—the last link with the past, the farthest extension of his future. The future of Camp Good Days and Special Times would be riding on how Gary Mervis would finish the summer.

Some of those close to Teddi's story were there that night, before Camp opened. Each returned that third year for their own reasons and the result of their own reflections.

"Why did I come back?" Muggs Register said matter-of-factly. "There wouldn't be any reason for Teddi, if I didn't." Polly Schwensen was having a difficult time when she arrived. She was assigned to the same cabin as the year before, when Teddi was there. Polly asked Muggs to stay with her in the cabin that night but Muggs had declined saying: "I'm living with the fear that at some moment during the next two weeks Teddi's death is going to hit me and I'm going to fall on my face and not be able to get up."

Later that same night, as the sun began to set, Skip DeBiase went out to the dock with his son, Alex. Together they broke worms into small pieces and cast them out onto the waters.

The next morning, through breakfast and lunch, the campgrounds were unusually quiet. Some of the veterans remarked about it. Though nobody said so out loud, a few felt it wasn't going to work, that something irretrievably had changed.

Counselors and staff walked alone or in small groups. And even in groups they seemed to be turned inward, as if thinking or maybe even praying. They seemed nervous. Others seemed to be storing their last bit of energy for the exhausting time ahead. A few worried about the size of their own courage.

Then a voice boomed over the loudspeaker, hammering home the message: "Five minutes to go!" And it was then that they seemed to forget their doubts, nervousness and fear—or overcame them—for they came running. They came out of the dining hall, the cabins, and from the beachfront. It looked like a tidal wave; a tidal wave of hope and commitment. Fingers clicked, people jumped up and down cheering, and clapping and crying. Crossroads the Clown blew on his horn over and over again, with wild abandon, gleeful and perhaps grateful he could do something with the excitement and love he was feeling.

The first bus then crept slowly onto the Camp's playing field. "The Olym-

Though Gary Mervis still talked and joked with kids, counselors, reporters, and anyone else who needed him, he seemed quieter than usual, more inward. Late at night, when nearly everyone else was asleep, he could be seen sitting on the front porch of the cabin, staring out into the darkness.

Nurses seemed to be the brunt of everyone's humor and jokes, campers and counselors alike. They made nurse Anne Cameron challenge Nurse Practitioner Mary Ellen Dasson to a banana-eating contest. Later, they blindfolded Barb Fredette and made her eat assorted foodstuffs from a pan. Barb was doing fine until she picked up a sausage link and the kids started shouting, "Worm! Worm!"

Sande Macaluso, watching events unfold and friendships form, would say, "You know, I'd like nothing better than to see this Camp close because they found a cure. But I'd want it to stay open forever if they didn't." Big tough guys like Ron Baldassare, a lightweight boxing champ in the Army, could be seen patiently and gently tying the shoes of a little girl, his hands the size of her head. Charlie Fornataro, a security-alarm specialist growing up in a tough city neighborhood, had become "Apples" the clown.

LaVerne Haley, probably suffering more in three years than most suffer in a lifetime, pointed at a child with a missing limb.

"What happened to her?" he asked his counselor.

"She has bone cancer," the counselor answered. "That's why her arm is gone."

He shook his small, frail head slowly from side to side. "That's too bad, isn't it?" he said.

Milly Wolf, the first head of the Teddi Project committee, would pretend she was jealous because one of her favorite young male campers was talking to another female counselor. "Sure, you leave me for a blonde," Milly teased. "But I only have this gray hair because I'm married to an older man."

The boy looked up. He was deadly earnest. "I don't care if you have green hair," he told Milly. "I'd love you anyway."

Later, the writer would learn that Milly had lost a child to cancer.

Toward the end of that first week, in the morning and as campers and counselors passed by the main cabin on their way to breakfast, each was surprised by the huge brown Teddy Bear sitting in a chair on the front porch. The bear wore a Camp Good Days and Special Times sweatshirt and cap. A note was attached to it and it read, in part:

> . . . I want to be the Camp mascot because it is a wonderful place to live. If you keep me, make certain promises. Make certain I'm always there to greet the buses when they arrive, and when they leave. Take me with you on Camp activities and give me a new Camp button each year. Always make certain that the campers and staff give me a lot of love. I would like to sit on the porch and greet each new person with love.

On the medical history form, also attached, the bear requested Dr. Klemperer as its physician.

"Talent Night" at Camp, an extraordinary event, is maybe the most significant in each of the two weeks. Often with their counselors, the children put on skits and sing songs and sometimes tell what they want and need and would miss most when the time comes for them to leave this earth.

Such was the case with LaVerne Haley, who at the end of the first week of Camp, hobbled onto the stage on Talent Night with the help of his counselor. LaVerne, often cranky and downright irascible at times, was also a hero to many because the doctors kept telling him he didn't have long to live and he kept on living anyway.

As LaVerne slowly made his way to the center of the stage the hall erupted—people clapped and cheered and stomped their feet and wouldn't let LaVerne speak or move. Then they rose to their feet, some shouting and some holding back their tears. Everyone, it seemed, was telling this little guy they loved him and that when he died they would miss him.

LaVerne, wearing a beret and red sweater and with a small guitar slung around his shoulders, seemed non-plussed by the exhibition of such emotion. Then the house grew quiet. For a second it seemed as though LaVerne was uncertain what he was to do next, or had forgotten the words to what he wanted to sing. Everyone waited, patiently. At Camp Good Days and Special Times there is no room for jeering or ridicule. The writer crossed his fingers.

After a whispered conversation with his counselor, LaVerne began strumming his guitar, saying the same line over and over again. Those present heard it differently. Some thought he was saying, "Don't take my *love* away." To others, it sounded more like: "Don't take my *life* away."

Nurse Practitioner Mary Ellen Dasson got up and moved to the back of the room, her eyes reddening. Dr. Klemperer took out his handkerchief. He said he always carried one with him because doctors had to sometimes cry.

Later, they would call Dr. Klemperer to the stage, and the place would erupt again. School was starting and he had to go back to the West Virginia medical college where he taught. As he stood there, the speech was going through his head: how he would tell the aspiring doctors about his time at Camp, with children with cancer, and how much they had taught him about living and loving. He would tell his aspiring doctors that medicine was both a science and an art, and that study, apprenticeship, and practice would prepare them to treat the body but that they must also come to understand the heart—their own and those they minister to. He would tell them all to carry a handkerchief with them, and if they didn't use it from time to time, they better think twice about becoming a doctor.

Dr. Klemperer used a handkerchief one final time at Camp. One of the last people to say good-bye to him was Skip DeBiase. He started to reach out his hand but Skip would have none of it. He kissed the doctor instead.

"When you're Italian and you love somebody you kiss them," he told the man.

Perhaps the hardest time for Gary and Sheri Mervis came on Monday, the second week of Camp. During that first week there had been a beautiful child who resembled Teddi greatly—Teddi the first year she had gone to Camp, when she was healthy and alert. So much did the child resemble Teddi that Judge Tony Bonadio, one of the volunteers, mistakenly began to wave to her, thinking it was Teddi again. But the second week of Camp brought a girl who reminded nearly everyone of Teddi of the year before, when Teddi had trouble speaking and walking, and when the decline was clear.

When Sheri first saw this girl arrive, she immediately turned away, walking off by herself. She removed her glasses with one hand and brought the other to her eyes. Gary met the girl that first night after flag raising. She was in the golf cart seated next to nurse Mary Schwartz.

"Hi, I'm Gary Mervis," he said, sticking out his hand.

She could barely stretch hers out far enough.

Gary asked where she was from and and what her name was and she told him. She also told him she had had a birthday the day before.

The nurse asked what she got for presents and the child answered, with some effort, that she had received a Pac Man quilt, a necklace, and a few other things.

Gary was nodding. "So you just had a birthday," he was saying. "How old are you now?"

She told him she was twelve, the same age Teddi was when she died.

"Have you ever been to Disney World?" Gary asked.

The child shook her head no.

Gary asked her if she liked Mickey Mouse and the child smiled and said she did. "Would you like to go to Disney World?" he asked, and she continued smiling. Eagerly yet softly she said, "Yes, I would like that."

"We're going to make sure you get to Disney World when Camp is over," he told her.

A counselor drove the child down to dinner, and Gary and the nurse began walking toward the infirmary. Nurse Schwartz was to go on duty.

"What does she have?" Gary asked, not looking at her.

"A brain tumor," answered Nurse Schwartz.

At the infirmary Gary looked over the girl's medical record. Attached to the cover sheet, at the top, was a picture of her before the treatments had started, before the baldness and weight gain and all the other side effects occurring prior to death. Nurse Shwartz watched as Gary got up from his chair and strolled alone along the beach.

Meanwhile, at dinner, Sheri watched as Muggs—who had taken over as counselor to the girl—got up with the child midway through dinner. The girl had to go to the bathroom. It was then Sheri made a decision that would affect her own life, and the future of the Camp, for the two had become intertwined now for the Mervises. Terrible as it was, Sheri honestly did not want to see or touch this child because it was like being with Teddi all over again, the Teddi who was dying. Yet she also knew that the child didn't deserve her coldness or indifference; that this was not Teddi but a child who had come and who had every right to the attention and love that the Camp held out as its promise.

Sheri rose from the table and after several minutes the child returned, Muggs wheeling her in, Sheri doting over her—as she would for the remainder of the Camp, sometimes to the chagrin of a counselor or two who thought the girl was being spoiled. Sheri had heard it all and seen it all before. There's no way you can ever spoil a child, no way you can give a child who's about to die the love they would have received with a lifetime of living.

Kim seemed to be having an easier time of it than Tod those two weeks. She seemed to be without inhibitions, as was evident when she was told that an especially handsome but shy boy was not participating in many of the Camp's events.

With the adults gathered together at a meeting in the dining hall, Kim commandeered the Camp microphone. "Will all available female campers and counselors please report to the main office! Will all available female campers and counselors report to the main office!" After they all had arrived she set about introducing them to the shy boy who stood there red-faced, shaking hands and smiling.

Tod worked and played hard those two weeks. He was growing up fast. One afternoon as he was sitting on the steps of his cabin a nurse walked by. She asked him what was wrong. "You know, this place is scary," he said. "A lot of these kids are going to end up like my sister."

Later, on a bus ride, the little girl who looked a lot like Teddi—and who for some reason had gravitated to Tod—accidentally bumped him in the nose. It made Tod's eyes water. "Big boys don't cry," she said to him.

He smiled. "Big boys are only allowed to cry when they lose in wrestling or someone passes away," he told her.

The Camp really had two endings. At the end of the first week about half of those due to leave departed. The other half, after checking with their parents, stayed for the second week, too. Counselors volunteered to stay on; Sheri ordered more pasta.

During the Camp's first ending, the writer wandered through the crowd jotting notes about gestures, expressions, and even overheard conversations. He then saw the mascot Teddy Bear and kneeled beside it, observing the Camp's touching farewell from the same place Teddi had viewed it the year before.

LaVerne wandered through the crowd of hugging and tears by himself, heading toward the mascot bear. Then he climbed into the chair, making for a tight fit with the bear. Finally, he turned and said: "Do you mind if I call you uncle?"

This was the first time he talked to the writer, and the writer was glad for the opportunity. "That would be okay," he said to the boy.

Then LaVerne asked if he could see the pen.

The writer tried to explain to the boy that he needed the pen in order to record the details of what was happening so he could use them later in a book he was writing about Teddi and the Camp. LaVerne wasn't impressed and so the writer gave him his pen—which LaVerne immediately began to disassemble. He couldn't get it put back together again and so the writer helped him. LaVerne then asked for a piece of paper.

While LaVerne drew on the paper, the writer tried to imprint upon his memory what remained of the Camp's first good-bye. Then a boy-clown came up to the chair. The boy-clown never talked in costume, nor disclosed his identity, but it was believed he was a child with cancer, too.

LaVerne looked up. "If I grow up," he told the boy, "I want to be a clown, too." And then the two boys kissed, on the lips, tenderly and without embarrassment. For some reason the writer thought of the little boy who had come for Teddi that previous Autumn, when the trees were bare and hope slim.

LaVerne folded his drawing, put a heart on it, and then handed it to the writer. The writer thanked him and, without blinking an eye or further acknowledgment, LaVerne drifted into the maelstrom of people still awaiting the boarding of the buses.

Slipping LaVerne's folded paper into his pocket, the writer immediately began writing down what he remembered, and what he was seeing. It was several days before he emptied his pockets to find the drawing. He unfolded it and found that LaVerne had drawn the writer's face—beard, baseball cap, and all. And the writer smiled at this special gift, thinking that maybe LaVerne was trying to welcome him into and inside the strange, unforgettable world of children with cancer, telling him that he was both writing the story and now part of the story as well.

As the second week of Camp drew to a close, there was again a "Talent Night." Dr. Harvey Cohen, from Strong Memorial Hospital, had replaced Dr. Klemperer as the Camp's medical director that second week. A big bear of a man, Cohen rose from his seat midway through that night's performances and sat in the back of the hall, his face hidden by the shadows.

Sitting next to him, the hall quiet now, the writer asked if the doctor would mind telling him what he was thinking.

"I was thinking about a story I saw on M*A*S*H once," he said. "A young soldier had died and Hawkeye was feeling pretty terrible. The old doctor took him aside and told him there were only two rules he had to remember. The first is that the young die. And the second is that you can't change rule number one. I was thinking about that."

The Camp's second ending was even more strained and powerful than the first. A whole year of planning, waiting, and giving was now at an end. There aren't many happy good-byes, but at Camp Good Days and Special Times the experience is devastating.

The sky was in conflict that morning as the buses waited, and campers and counselors scurried around trying to match clothes with people, and keep too busy to notice the rumbling tide of emotions rising inside. The sun was still definitely summer's. It was warm and bright. But the clouds were Autumn's—leaving the air chilled and the ground with large dark shadows as they meandered passed the sun. The chill and shadows caused people to look up, wondering how long before the sun would warm them and the ground again.

It was a gentle time. The hugs—the kisses and pats on the back—were the kind you would give a friend you liked a lot, someone you knew you might not see again for a very long time. You could see people hanging onto one another in twos and threes, swaying.

Gary Mervis held up a little boy who was crying. "You going to be okay?" he asked, trying to comfort the child. Gary's brother Bob, standing next to him, let out a deep sigh. Sheri helped the child who looked like Teddi onto her bus and quickly walked away, her back to everyone, taking off her glasses as she left. Kim Mervis was weeping openly and without reservation. Her brother Tod loaded sleeping bags and carried those who could not walk, trying to comfort people even though tears were falling from his eyes, too.

Veteran journalists were there, people who covered car crashes, murders, and other tragedies, and they seemed speechless, without purpose, standing in the center of what seemed like a profound spiritual experience. Dr. Cohen wandered through the crowd, eyes reddened, hugging everyone in sight—including the writer. "It's wonderful, isn't it?" he said, before moving on. Someone else in the crowd could be heard saying, "I didn't think things like this happened on earth."

Charlie Fornataro held up the mascot Teddy Bear, waving its arms. "Say good-bye to Teddy," he was calling out, and children ran over and climbed off the bus to give the bear, and Charlie, a final hug and kiss good-bye.

As the last of the children climbed aboard the buses and the engines started, the campsite grew markedly quiet. Counselors and staff still waved and called out final "I love you's" and good-byes, but the sound, and the experience of Camp, had definitely turned in a different direction. They themselves looked a little lost now, a little incomplete, as if part of them was leaving along with the buses. Some seemed to be wandering around looking for a final handshake or a hug.

"Crossroads the Clown" checked the tires and mirrors of every bus before it left. And as it pulled out of the playing field, the clown would run alongside it, as if wanting to stay with it all the way home. But each time he ran alongside a bus, he would bump into a tree and be stopped, legs and arms flailing every which way. It was absurd to watch, and yet it also seemed fitting, for there are few things on earth as absurd as the death of children.

The leaves at the top of the particular tree that stopped him, a maple tree, had already begun to turn a bright crimson. Autumn came early to the Adirondacks, and its leaves would feel the cold and leave much sooner than trees elsewhere.

The writer, sitting on the bleachers, watched the counselors and staff walk back to the cabins and dining hall. The campground was silent now, except for the wind. For two full weeks children laughed, shouted, sang, cheered, and told secrets, and now it was all quiet.

Just then a hawk came into view, flying over the road which the buses had taken. It circled and soared, like a silent soul, wondering, it seemed, why this strange silence had descended over the land.

The Indians who once roamed the Adirondacks, and named them, believed that it meant good luck when a hawk flew overhead before a difficult journey.

PART IV

Epilogue

33

A Place in the World

That difficult third summer and the year that followed began to produce evidence that the Camp Good Days and Special Times organization was not only here to stay but would make a sizable difference in the lives of children with cancer. Today, it is the largest organization of its kind for children with cancer in the world.

The summer component of the Camp itself expanded in terms of the number of children attending, and the numbers volunteering. That first summer of 1980, the Camp hosted sixty-three children. By the summer of 1989, more than 700 campers and 900 volunteers were in attendance. In its first decade, the Camp has been the summer home for more than 3,300 children from all over upstate New York and beyond.

Though it was originally designed as a residential program for children with cancer between the ages of seven to seventeen, founder Gary Mervis believed there ought to be something done for children even younger. As a result, the Camp introduced a special four-day summer day program for children with cancer between the ages of four and seven years. It is called the Junior Camp Good Days.

Understanding the special needs of families coping with cancer expanded each year, and with it so did Camp programs and plans.

Siblings of children with cancer have unique fears and problems, and Camp Good Days and Special Times has set aside summer time for them as well. The idea was inspired by Teddi's own siblings, Tod and Kim, who feared they or their offspring would develop cancer. Experience also showed that siblings would sometimes feel guilty because they think they may have caused the cancer or the pain their siblings have to go through. Often they feel left out. Gary Mervis refers to the siblings of children with cancer as "the forgotten ones."

Brothers and Sisters Together, or BEST, was spawned to give siblings of children with cancer an opportunity for summer fun. During their summer stay, an effort is also made to help them understand cancer's affect on their own lives.

Camp Good Days has also established Moms 'n Pops, an ongoing program for parents of children with cancer. Its purpose is to give mothers and fathers a break from their worry and demands on their time. It provides them as well with an opportunity to share their feelings and fears with others.

A special quality of the summer component of Camp Good Days and Special Times is that it is staffed by volunteers. People come because they want to come: the medical team, the kitchen crew, the trained counselors and specialists donate their time every summer. These volunteers, when they leave Camp after the summer is over, return to their workplaces and communities with different feelings and understandings about children with cancer. In this way, too, the wall of ignorance and indifference with respect to childhood cancer gets chipped away.

The Camp has also begun to witness the return of former campers who now come back as counselors. Gary Mervis estimates their number to be at about 15 percent of the total volunteer staff. He believes that number will grow as more and more former campers survive their cancer. These former campers also provide inspiration for younger campers: They're living examples of kids who beat the odds.

A "good" problem for the Camp is there are many more applicants who apply to be volunteers than the Camp can take. Mervis estimates that about half of the more than 700 who applied as camp counselors for the 1989 season had to be turned down. Though Mervis said it's tough to turn down so many good people, there simply wasn't room for them at the Camp. Those selected to be volunteers represent a variety of occupations and ages, from blue-collar workers to judges, doctors and lawyers—nurses, students, mothers, fathers and even grandparents volunteer. They come from all over the country and as far away as Australia.

Over the years, the summer component of the Camp Good Days and Special Times organization has served as a model to other such summer camps for children with cancer in the United States and around the world. When Camp Good Days and Special Times first began there were only four such camps in the United States; now there are eighty similar organizations in the United States. These camps have collectively joined together to share information and ideas in a national organization called COCA—Childhood Oncology Camps of America.

But Camp Good Days and Special Times has expanded in several other ways as well and it is this feature which makes it the largest and most comprehensive organization of its kind in the world.

One mainstay of the early years of the organization is the Teddi Project. Named after Teddi Mervis, this volunteer program was originally structured to fulfill the last wish of terminally ill children with cancer. Now all terminally ill children may apply, and more than 200 children have participated over the years. These children and their families have gone to Disney World, to Hawaii, or even to visit grandparents from out of town. Some, such as Clarence "Huggy" Pettway, even got a chance to meet his favorite celebrity, Bill Cosby. Their relationship received national attention.

Huggy, his mother, and sister flew to New York City to watch a rehearsal of the Cosby Show, a trip paid out of the Teddi Project. Huggy gave Cosby a sweatshirt printed with the camp's name. Later, upon hearing that Huggy's condition was worsening, Cosby called the child to tell him that he was going to wear the sweatshirt on his show. Cosby also took the opportunity to invite Huggy to be part of an upcoming Cosby episode, but Huggy died shortly afterward.

After Huggy's death and in one show's epilogue, Cosby mentioned to his actress wife the names of the people he wanted to invite to his birthday party. It was to be a small party, he said, and he wanted only special friends to be there. One of the names he mentioned on the air was that of Clarence "Huggy" Pettway.

Part of the reason the Teddi Project has been able to expand in several ways is the result of the fund-raising efforts of the students at St. John Fisher College. A small liberal arts college in Rochester, New York, the College annually hosts a twenty-four-hour dance marathon to raise money specifically for the Teddi Project. About a fourth of the entire College participates—mainly students—but also including Fisher's President, the Dean, and others of the faculty and staff. Ironically, Gary Mervis has often said that St. John Fisher College, down the road from the Mervis home, was where Teddi would have liked to have gone had she lived. The writer runs the marathon each year. Now part of the story, Fisher is where he is a teacher.

Along with the Teddi Project, Camp Good Days and Special Times has pioneered other programs which have made it more than a summer facility. One such program is Childhood U.S.A. (Understanding/Support and Assistance), designed for children who have a parent with cancer. The program's emphasis is on keeping the lines of communication open between child and parent and in providing recreational and other activities in which both may participate. Additionally, Childhood U.S.A. offers a bereavement program to help children cope with the death of a parent.

Taking a lesson from Teddi's experience with school, Camp Good Days and Special Times offers a workshop series for teachers and school nurses. Called "Cancer in the Classroom," the program is designed to acquaint educational professionals with the disease of cancer itself and the unique world inhabited by children with cancer.

Camp Good Days has established a program which matches newly diagnosed cancer patients with young volunteers who have had the disease for at least one year and who are now in remission. Gary Mervis remembered how isolated Teddi had been and how difficult it was for her to talk about her cancer, even to parents, cognizant of the pain such conversations caused.

An additional factor leading to the program's birth is the fact that more and more children diagnosed as having cancer survive. These children, Mervis felt, need somebody to talk with about making their way back into the mainstream.

According to Dr. Harvey Cohen, chief of the division of Pediatric Hematology-Oncology at the University of Rochester Medical School, as many as 60 percent of all children who are diagnosed as having cancer will now survive. About 12,500 new cases of pediatric cancer are diagnosed each year in the United States—and between 2,000 and 3,000 children die.

Camp Good Days has also established a very active Explorer Post for children over thirteen with cancer. The post meets monthly throughout the school year. Besides participating in traditional scouting activities, these teens also do service projects throughout the year. The John Wolf Pediatric Cancer Information Center can be found at the Camp's Rochester headquarters. The Center maintains up-to-date information and reference material for public use. The Camp also throws several large holiday parties for all children from the Camp's programs—their parents, volunteers and all key people who throughout the year help the Camp in a variety of ways.

The Camp changed its summer location from New York's Adirondack region to the state's Finger Lakes. From 1981 to 1988, it rented its summer facilities and had to work around other camping schedules—sometimes using as many as five different camps. The situation created enormous logistical problems.

The number of campers wanting to attend each year was increasing, and some had to be placed on waiting lists. Parents had to be kept up to date regarding the new summer location of the camp and camping dates. The Camp staff and volunteers had to set up the Camp each year, coordinating the delivery of its own medical and recreational supplies and renovating campgrounds to make them accessible for the physically handicapped. Once Camp was over, the operation repeated itself in reverse, with the additional problem of storage between sessions.

These problems motivated the Camp's founder and organization to launch a $1.7 million drive to purchase and renovate a permanent recreational facility for Camp Good Days and Special Times, Inc. A bonus to the drive was the entrance of actress Candice Bergen as chairperson of the drive. Bergen came to Rochester often, donating her time and talent for public service announcements, and to do a lengthy fund-raising video for the drive.

As was true so many times before, Gary Mervis went out on the campaign trail again, this time trying to convince others of the need for a permanent facility. "With a permanent home," he'd say, over and over again and again, "we'll be able to concentrate fully on the quality of our programs and not worry about the logistics of setting up and tearing down five times a summer."

He'd tell them of his dream to have a place specially designed to meet the needs of campers with cancer. "Besides having plenty of room for everybody," he'd tell them, eyes beaming with his dream, "everything will be accessible to handicapped campers. Our infirmary will be permanently equipped for camping—and cancer—emergencies." And then he would conclude: "We'll be able to devote a whole summer to Good Days camping, and have a home for programs throughout the year."

The campaign to establish a permanent facility met its goal. As funds poured in, Camp Good Days purchased a site near the Keuka Lake village of Branchport and work began. The twenty-five acres already had existing buildings, but these had to be renovated and made handicap accessible, and new buildings were needed. In his unique way, Gary got business and labor unions to donate materials and their time in aiding in the construction and rennovation. A 2,500-square-foot dining hall was built. With donated time and materials, the $250,000 building was constructed for a cost to the Camp budget of only $50,000.

Camp Good Days and Special Times opened its permanent home, fittingly, on Memorial Day, 1989. "It's really been a dream come true," Gary Mervis told a reporter at the time, and indeed it was. Everything in the new facility was accessible to handicapped campers just as Gary had promised. There was even a handicapped-accessible swimming pool so that wheelchair bound children with cancer could go in the water. Kids with tubes placed into them, tubes which have to be kept clean, could now also enjoy the water. The new Camp had an infirmary specially designed to deal with camping and cancer emergencies. The new facility was big enough so that no child with cancer would have to be put on a waiting list.

As they had at previous camps, children still came in all stages of their cancer—those in complete remission and those who wouldn't make it much past the following Autumn. They come healthy looking; and they come without limbs and blind. As at previous camps, they ate as many hamburgers and ice cream sundaes as they wanted. They ate pizza from boxes, and at one supper they sat at tables with linens and silverware. Nearly 25,000 meals were served up at the new facility that first summer. Cooks from the U.S. Army Reserve 98th Division donated their services, as they had the previous seven years.

Children went canoeing, sailing, swimming, and played golf, basketball, softball, and volleyball. They went for hot-air balloon and seaplane rides and they tried their hand at Project Adventure—a ropes course designed to help build cooperation and trust.

The new Camp has tennis courts, horseback-riding facilities, a go-cart track, a nine-hole miniature golf course, horseshoe pits, and even its own "store" so that campers could spend camp coupons for small items. Youngsters danced to rock bands, walked nature trails, and sang around campfires. There was a camp horse to pet, and two camp dogs to play with.

A special part of the new Camp's opening was the tenth anniversary reunion of campers and counselors from the first Camp. One former camper who flew in from Brownsville, Texas, told a reporter: "Ten years ago, most of us kids couldn't even count on what would happen to us next week. Ten years was something you wouldn't even dare think about." Another former camper returned with his two young children. Though doctors had predicted that his chances of survival were 1 in 100,000, he lived to prove that odds could be beaten. Doctors also had said radiation would leave him unable to father children. Still another returning camper was now in her second year of nursing school.

Those who came for the reunion also conducted a brief memorial service for the more than two dozen others who had died. They planted a rose bush at the base of a statue which greets visitors to the Camp. The statue is more like a tower, emblazened with teddy bears and laughing children. Two hands reach skyward from the top of the tower, clutching a string that holds a trinity of brass balloons. During the service they sang "The Rose" and each poured a small glass of water on the newly planted rose bush.

The Camp truly became international that first summer at its new facility. Six youngsters from Jerusalem, Israel, were invited to take part in two, one-week sessions of Camp Good Days. An Israeli doctor, meeting with Dr. Harvey Cohen at the University of Rochester, heard about Camp Good Days and thought it would be wonderful if children from his own country could come and have the experience.

The Camp also opened its doors that first summer at its new home to children whose parents or siblings are AIDS victims. Sixteen came that summer, their identities a closely guarded secret. The announcement of the move met with opposition from the local community, and Gary Mervis received hate mail and anonymous phone calls. "It put quite a strain on my family," he said.

Mervis met with members of the community and kept lines of communication open at his office for anyone upset or worried about the new AIDS camp. He said he wanted to give these children a chance to befriend someone who can understand what they are going through; to distribute information and answer children's questions honestly; and to give these children a chance to have fun during what can be a very tense time. For Mervis, the last reason was as important as any.

"A serious illness can cause the family income to go down and some of the kids may have even just lost a parent or sibling," Gary told a Rochester reporter. "It gives these kids a chance to stand up at school in September and tell about some fun things they did over the summer."

During the past decade, Camp Good Days and Special Times and its innovative programs have served as models for other pediatric oncology camps from Vermont to California in the United States, as well as in Montreal, New Zealand, and Japan. The Camp's national recognition, because of its accomplishments and positive impact, has attracted the media—as well as politicians, sports stars, and other celebrities.

The Camp has been written about in popular publications such as *McCall's*, *USA Today*, and *The New York Times*, and major medical journals such as *Oncology Times*, *Cancer Today*, and *Cancer Nursing*. It's also been the subject of television news and documentary programs.

Teddi herself, when she was alive, sat on President Gerald Ford's lap and received an autographed picture; a group of campers later visited the Reagan White House and had their picture taken with the ex-President and his wife. New York Governor Mario and Matilda Cuomo, HUD Secretary Jack Kemp, and others have recognized the Camp's importance and taken note of the changes in attitudes toward childhood cancer and the part Camp Good Days and Special Times has played in that change.

Coaching legends in basketball and football have turned up for events which benefit Camp Good Days and Special Times. Big East coaches such as Syracuse's Jim Boeheim, Georgetown's John Thompson, Villanova's Rollie Massimino, and Seton Hall's P. J. Carlesimo have come to Rochester to help raise money for Good Days programs and have done free PSAs to further advance the Camp's cause.

While the Camp has a permanent facility, and some of its programs still endure, Camp Good Days and Special Times is an evolving type organization quick to recognize and meet new challenges—always planning, preparing, and breaking new ground. For example, the Camp recently bought a home in Florida because most children say they want to visit Disney World as part of the Teddi Project. Mervis believed such a residence would be less expensive and more convenient than hotel rooms, and could be stocked with special provisions to meet the needs of cancer patients. "It would cut the costs of these trips to Disney World for families by 40 or 50 percent," he says. Gary Mervis also hopes to extend education and support programs to families in the Orlando area after the residence is established.

There are other challenges in the decade ahead, says Mervis. He hopes better understanding of childhood cancer will come. "Childhood cancer is different from adult cancer, and we really don't know why some children are predisposed to it and others aren't."

Mervis also believes that the first generation of long-term survivors of childhood cancer lies ahead and with it new problems and challenges. "What kind of career opportunities will be open to them?" Mervis asks. "Will they be welcome in the military? Be able to join police and fire departments? Will employers refuse to hire them because they don't want to invest in somebody who might die early, or might be sick a lot or even make others in the workplace feel uncomfortable?"

But Mervis sees dealing with children of AIDS—those who have it or come from a family which has it—as the major challenge of the next decade. "These kids come from the poorest of the poor, have no political clout, and the issue is how to provide for a quality of life for these kids. AIDS kids are at a place where childhood cancer was when we first started. People fear it's contagious, or it's something they can even pick up at the house of a victim. These kids are isolated from the rest of the world."

As Gary reflects on the enormity of time and effort that went into the building of Camp Good Days and Special Times, he talks about the toll it has taken on him personally, and on his family. "I haven't taken a vacation in 25 years," he says wistfully. "I'd like to drop a fishline in the waters of the St. Lawrence River in the next decade—and I'd like to be able to take my grandchildren, when they arrive, to the zoo or a ballgame."

Tod Mervis now works at the Camp full-time, taking over many of the tasks his father once performed. Kim is a nursing student and plans on spending her working life attending to the medical needs of children. Sheri Mervis had begun to separate from the Camp more and more over the years, searching for new interests and goals, and finally separated from Gary himself. Catastrophic illness is devastating on family life and the Mervises did not escape its impact.

Gary Mervis, once a large person, has shed some 70 pounds today, like a man starting anew—and in many ways he is. He's more reflective now, less impatient, even more spiritual. "I'm not a very religious person," he said, "but I believe in God. And I pray that my family understands I tried to do right by them. I also pray that I always do what's right for Camp Good Days and Special Times."

What began as one man's desire to see that his terminally ill daughter was modestly happy and comforted has impacted positively on the lives of thousands of children who were once ignored and largely absent from life itself. What began from frustration and anguish has challenged and changed the consciousness of the common person, celebrities, politicians, corporate heads, and journalists and writers throughout the northeast—and indeed the nation.

The Camp Good Days and Special Times story is one of triumph and courage. The story has been an enormous practical success. It also has pushed the human heart to redefine what it knows about hope—and to understand the costs of truly loving.

Afterword

A decade has gone by since *For the Love of Teddi* was first published. I have always felt, as the writer of this story, that Gary Mervis's love for his daughter is manifest by the Camp itself: its mission, its passion to reduce suffering among children, its commitment to the sanctity of life itself. Camp Good Days and Special Times is as big and important as one father's love—a poignant reminder to us all about turning tragedy into good in the world.

In 1990, when this book was first published, Camp Good Days and Special Times expanded its operations to the children and families of Central Florida. It maintains an office in Tampa, Florida and rents various camps in the area. Going to Disney World still remains a foremost dream of terminally ill children, and the Camp, with facilities in Florida, is better able to accommodate the special needs of these children and their families. Camp Good Days also purchased and developed its own recreational facility on the shore of Keuka Lake, in Branchport, New York.

The Camp continues to bring out the best in people. New programs, new volunteers, and new children to help prompted the need for more space. The Rochester & Finger Lakes Chapters of Allied Building and Construction Trades pitched in and built a beautiful new Headquarters and Volunteer Training Facility for the Camp in Mendon, New York, a small town near Rochester. Nearly all of the labor and half the materials were donated.

Throughout the early 1990s, a series of sports dinners were held in Rochester, New York, hosted by Gary's long-time friend, Pete Pavia. Pavia, an NCAA Division I basketball official, was diagnosed with cancer the same month in 1979 as Teddi. After surgery, he remained cancer-free for many years, continued his officiating, and helped bring sports celebrities into town for the dinner.

From the world of basketball, these included Patrick Ewing, John Thompson, John Calipari, Rollie Massimino, PJ Carlesimo, Jim Boeheim, and Rick Barnes. Washington Redskins notables Russ Grimm, Don Warren, Mark Rypien, and Wayne Sevier also came. Unfortunately, Pete lost his battle to cancer. One final dinner was held in his honor and the monies raised went into the construction of a new, beautiful recreational facility at the Keuka Lake campsite—The Pavia Pavilion.

To me, Gary has always been masterful at making connections between what the world is and what the world should be. In 1993, the Center for Disease Control in Atlanta announced that violence in America was a disease, and that without specific intervention, children from violent environments would become either victims or perpetrators. In response, Gary began the Sharing and Caring Program for children who have been affected by a homicide in their family. In addition to a week-long residential camping program, the children also take part in monthly recreational support programs.

Shortly after starting the Sharing and Caring Program, Jennifer Koon, a St. John Fisher College student, was senselessly and brutally murdered. Gary's ties to the college run deep: when Teddi got older, she wanted to go to school there; students annually host a 24-hour dance marathon for the Teddi Project; and Gary has been a long-time member of the college's football coaching staff. With the help of many in the community, Gary announced the establishment of the Partners Against Violence Everywhere (PAVE) Initiative. It was the Camp's contribution to the fight against crime and violence.

The PAVE Initiative now includes the Sharing and Caring Program as well as a new program—Creating Kids with Courage and Compassion. The latter consists of parenting seminars, a Community of Survivors support group, and community-wide memorial services. The PAVE Initiative was instrumental in helping bring Project Exile to Rochester—an anti-gun program modeled after the one in Richmond, Virginia. Gary serves as the Chairman for the Project Exile Advisory Board, which consists of federal, state, and local law enforcement personnel, the U.S. Attorney's Office, the District Attorney's Office, government officials, clergy, and local business leaders. After just one year of operation, the homicide rate in Rochester slumped to the lowest it had been in fourteen years.

Teddi's two siblings, Tod and Kim, grew up, married, and had children of their own. Tod and his wife Margie have three children: Mary Louise, Shane, and Theodore. Tod continues to work for Camp Good Days as the Safety Director and Project Adventure Ropes Course Instructor. Kim married Tim Roach and the couple have two daughters, Ryan and Delaney. Kim is a school nurse and Tim works as a school psychologist.

Gary married Wendy Bleier on June 10, 1995. Performing the ceremony was Teddi's priest, Father David Ambuske. The service was held at his small Anglican Church in Webster, New York—home of the memorial service to Teddi. The reception was held at the Convention Center in Downtown Rochester with 400 of their "closest friends" attending! Gary and Wendy currently reside in Pittsford, New York with their two dogs, Zaharis, a Rottweiler, and Jordyn, an English bulldog. Wendy is a physical education teacher and coach in the Rush-Henrietta School District. She has become very involved in helping Gary run Camp Good Days, especially during the summer, when she serves as Camp Director.

With Wendy's guidance and dedication, the Women's Oncology Program was introduced in 1996. Since its inception, more than 400 women dealing with cancer have had the opportunity to experience the magic and spirit of Camp Good Days. The program received national attention from *Ladies' Home Journal* as well as being included in a five-part series on breast cancer on *Good Morning America*. The oncology program has expanded to Central Florida and plans are underway to make it year-round, with the addition of a Recreational Support Program for the women.

In 1997, the Camp Good Days and Special Times Foundation was established with the expressed goal of putting together a succession plan when the time comes for Gary to step down. The Foundation is trying to raise the necessary funds and build an endowment that will ensure that Camp Good Days will be around as long as there is a need for it.

I had always thought that Gary and I would grow old together, having coffee once in a while, being there for Fisher football, parenting our children into adulthood. But a new opportunity at the University of North Carolina in Wilmington lured me away. My heart still is with the Camp. And last year I was invited back for the annual St. John Fisher College dance marathon. I didn't know any of the faces of the students, but their spirit was the same as that first dance marathon in 1982, dedicated to helping children with life-threatening illness. I had one hard thing to do as the night ended, my old friend Gary beside me, and that was to tell them they were part of the spirit of giving that refused to die, and that I was leaving the marathon forever in their faithful hands.

Camp Good Days has completed 21 years of providing residential camping programs and year-round activities and events for children and families whose lives have been touched by cancer, HIV/AIDS, violence, and other life-threatening challenges. Times change, and the challenges that campers face in 1979–80 when this story began are not the same as today.

Because of better strides made in the detection and treatment of cancer, there are more long-term survivors. Yet these children face new challenges: the possibility of sterility as a result of treatment, cognitive learning disabilities, short-term memory loss, and a host of new problems associated with interpersonal relationships and employment. A new worry for children today is the fear and anxiety that the cancer will reappear.

Camp Good Days and Special Times is dedicated to continuing to be at the forefront and to provide any help necessary to the children and families it serves. This is reflected in Gary's personal vision, manifest by the Camp's mission statement: "To be internationally recognized as the premiere service organization that enriches the lives of children, adults and families who are touched by cancer, AIDS, violence and other life challenges."

About the Author

LOU BUTTINO is Professor of Communication Studies at the University of North Carolina at Wilmington. He is the author of three books, scores of articles and feature stories, and more than twenty documentaries. He has received numerous academic fellowships and awards, including the award for distinguished scholarship from both St. John Fisher College and the University of North Carolina at Wilmington. Dr. Buttino has earned state, national, and international honors for his documentary work and he has appeared in the ESPN documentary special "Fighting the Mob: The Story of Carmen Basilio." He has also earned national recognition for his screenplays, including most recently "Carmen Basilio! Basilio!"